WIN THE NAIL GAME

COMPETITION SUCCESS MADE SIMPLE

"A winner never gives up!"
With love,
Ela Loszczyk

ELA LOSZCZYK

WIN THE NAIL GAME
COMPETITION SUCCESS MADE SIMPLE

Published by NAIL EXPERTS ACADEMY LTD
info@nailexpertsacademy.com

CONTENTS

Part II
Competition day

Part III
After the competition

WHO'S ELA LOSZCZYK?

"I believe that to be happy and successful you should do what you love and always do your best."

I'm Ela Loszczyk, founder of **Nail Experts Academy** and author of the book, *Win the Nail Game – Competition success made simple,* which you're holding in your hands right now.

My goal is to help nail technicians realise their full potential so they can provide more effective, precise and consistent service to customers. Also, I seek to inspire them to grow strong and be successful in the nail industry by combining and putting their nail-care and marketing skills into practice.

It's my passion to teach them in a way that is simple to understand and with that end in view I've started the Nail Experts Academy and written this book. But, as you can imagine, nothing happens overnight; so let me tell you how it all started.

My dream was born...

I was born and raised in Poland. For most of my teenage life I wanted to be a policewoman. I just loved the idea of me chasing bad guys or working as a detective at the crime scene and connecting all the evidential dots to solve the case. That made me study it at the university for three years to earn my bachelor's degree. I also did my masters but in social work and prisoner rehabilitation, as that was the only option available at that time. In the first of two years of my studies at the second university, I realised that I was missing something and that working with prisoners would not be my dream job.

Life went on as usual for a vivacious girl like me. I was taking care of myself quite well. I made sure that I was well turned out and that I paid attention to my physical attributes although I was not a beauty-freak. Then something happened. For the first time in 2005, I had my nails done for my wedding. I really liked it and wanted to do the nails myself although acrylic liquid made me sick at that time. I thought this was so simple that I didn't need to do any course! So I bought some stuff on ebay and started with myself. Soon I realised I couldn't get it quite the same way as my technician did while working on my nails, and was wondering why my brush went super hard after several uses.. Not giving up, I decided to treat my mum! While I was preparing her nails — filing them as much as possible — she complained about burning sensation around her nails and kept saying they felt quite sensitive. Ignoring her complaints I continued until I ended up over-filing one. And that was the moment when I decided to do a nail course.

I did it. I enrolled on a two-week-long pricey training course as I thought it to be the best one. I was wrong. The trainer wasn't helping me at all as she was busy with her own clients and business. Clearly, it wasn't the best choice and it left me with a huge disappointment. I knew I was missing the basics and nothing was fully explained. Incidentally, around that time, something important happened that completely changed my life and career plans. While on that course, I discovered what I really wanted to do. I wanted to teach! I promised myself that I would do it one day no matter what and that my students would never be treated the way I had been. My dream was born!

But here was the reality...

In 2006, I came to Edinburgh, Scotland with my husband Lukasz. We didn't want to live like our parents who had spent most of their life in Poland. As a young newly married couple we sought adventure; and wanted to discover new cultures, learn new things and try a different lifestyle. No friends, no close family members and grappling with the English language, I had to start from scratch. I had no idea how I was going to make my dream a reality, but I nurtured it all the same. I was practising on the only available model my husband. We spent many evenings on product application and removal.

I remember one night, when I was eight months pregnant and was practising "pink and white" (P&W) on Lukasz; I did five nails and then suddenly felt pain and thought I was in labour. I wasn't it was false alarm. "You don't expect me to go to the hospital with these nails, do you," he asked me. As I looked up, I found him biting acrylic off his nails!

The situation was comic. The whole point, however, is that you need to sacrifice something in order to become better at what you do. My goal was to give my future clients the best possible services and experience. I was hooked on nails. Doing them became my real passion. Once I really wanted to attend a workshop in Poland. My daughter Julia was 4 months' old then and I was breastfeeding her. She refused bottle-feeding; so leaving behind a hungry baby for three days wasn't an option. However, my desire to go was so strong that I took my mother — also living in the UK — along to babysit my daughter. She stayed with Julia in the hotel room and I was able to attend the workshop, although I missed a bit of it whenever I had to go upstairs to feed Julia. All that because of my passion for nails and my hunger for becoming a better nail tech.

I realised that if I wanted to teach the trade I had to learn it thoroughly. So I was attending more and more training courses, workshops and seminars that I'd carefully selected for myself. I'd been travelling abroad more often, investing a lot in my education and learning from top educators in the world. Even though I had to borrow money many times to attend those courses, I knew all this would help me fulfil my dream in a big way. It wasn't easy. During those difficult days I was toiling as a support worker with my little nail business a desk from Argos was set up for the purpose in my living room. I had to divide my time between work and Julia and had to try really hard to make money working long hours, two jobs and no holidays for years.

In 2009, I entered my first nail competition to test my skills. I wasn't really great at P&W then. To be honest, I was really bad and my smile lines looked quite grumpy. I remembered my educator from my second foundation course. She told me: "Ela stick to the nail art and forget about P&W. You're rubbish there." I listened to her and stayed focused on nail art for a while. But all my clients wanted P&W and I was doing several sets a day. Soon I realised that P&W was what people wanted and would have it over and over again, and that I'd better change my attitude and start liking it. I did so and discovered the real beauty of it. I fell in love with those perfectly filed shapes, crispy smile lines, C-curves and arches that I found on other people's nails but not mine. The more beautiful P&W's I saw, the more I wanted to do them and prove my educator wrong. I needed competition training. I did some research and went to Poland again for several days to be trained by Joanna, who had already won many competitions and I knew she would give me good tips and training. Then I started my preparations, practising twice a week for two months. When I heard the results of the competitions, I was very happy I came first in Sculpt P&W and second in Salon Nail Art.

Within the next three years I won many competitions and even held the title of Scottish and UK Nail Champion. Soon after I was invited to join various expert panels to judge nail competitions in the UK. My articles were published in the leading nail industry magazines in the UK and Poland, such as *Scratch, Your Nails, Paznokcie, Akademia Paznokcia,* etc. I'm very proud of being featured on the front covers of *Scratch* and *Paznokcie*. I also had a five-minute slot in "The Hour" show of STV television where I presented live a nail art to celebrate FIFA World Cup 2010.

In 2012, I entered my name in competitions organised by Scratch Stars. I was a finalist in the L&P Tech of the Year category and won the Gel Tech of the Year award. I couldn't attend the awards ceremony as my bonny baby boy was just born then. No regrets. In 2013 and 2014, I was a finalist again in the Nail Stylist category and the winner of L&P Tech of the Year award, which I'm very proud of as I absolutely love acrylic system and P&W.

My dream about teaching came true in 2008 when I became the only Master Educator for 25 countries for the company I was working with. I also became an International Educator teaching in countries such as UK, Ireland, Holland, Poland, Russia, and Malta.

I've trained hundreds of students and many of them run successful businesses by opening salons and nail bars, with a few of them even trading as mobile technicians. I've trained over 20 educators and led them as Education Director. These people are now into teaching using my structures and techniques. I was then running my own nail salon and was also the sole distributor of several nail brands in the UK.

I trained — and still do — nail technicians for competitions and many of them reached the podium even at the very beginning of their career.

The goals achieved, I started dreaming really big. I wanted to reach out to more students through high-quality online and offline (DVD) training courses to help them achieve their goals and benefit from my experience, no matter where they are in the world. This was the foundation and beginning of Nail Experts Academy. I've already recorded several classes, which are available on my website, and more courses and programmes will follow soon.

I'm known to deliver innovative and high-quality nail training courses in the industry and, importantly, **to help nail technicians get results fast!** My students learn from me practical skills and wisdom not only through live classes, but also through my articles, videos, programmes, online/offline training courses and books. You can check all my educational materials on **www.elaloszczyk.co.uk**. But because I don't know everything, I study and interview other experts and leaders from the nail and business industries in an effort to provide my students with up-to-date information and expertise. I feel that motivation and inspiration is important and really needed, so I do my weekly video-blog, packing it with lots of info and tips for my subscribers in order to keep them on track.

I believe that to be able to do great things and to realise all of your dreams you don't have to be unique or special. You just need to be clear on what you want and what your passion is, you need to be a go-getter. Everything can be learnt and everything can be achieved. The fact that you're starting small doesn't make YOU small. Every successful person started small somewhere.

I love to inspire people, inspire you, and show that you can really fulfil your desire only if you're passionate enough to do so and be in a fighting spirit. The best thing about it all is that it is never too late to start. There will always be a good time to change things around. If you've ever wanted to learn something new then do it, and I'm strictly speaking from experience! You need to keep learning, attending courses and staying up-to-date with trends to be in the reckoning. You'll have to do all this if you are really passionate about what you do. If you know someone you want to be trained by, then go and do it. There is no such thing as "too far", not in the twenty-first century. I know because I've travelled a lot and if I can learn something valuable from a person who's far away, there's always a way to make it happen.

Dream big. Reach your goals. Live your passion. We all live only once, so make sure you don't waste your time doing things you don't like. Focus on your purpose and live it. You're part of a great industry so make use of it while you can.

ABOUT THIS BOOK

For many years I've been competing in various nail championships and taking competition training courses. And for many years too, I had this nagging feeling that there's something missing. I wasn't sure what it was until one of my students told me she'd love to have a book about championships. It lit the bulb in my head at once!

I decided to write this book and inspire you not only to enter nail competitions, but also to do more than others to reach your goals, to push your boundaries and to never stop learning. Someone told me once that if we're not growing then we're dying. I do believe that and if my book becomes your inspiration and competition guide, then it has served its purpose.

This book is a collection of strategies that I've learned through experiences I gathered while taking part in competitions, doing training courses or sitting as judge on contests. I've also written down what I learnt from my students' struggles and success stories.

I realised that taking part in competitions was actually a game where every competitor was a player. We play against each other to the rules and try hard to earn valuable points. Your job as contestant is to play the game, make a minimum number of mistakes and score most. That's how you win it. I also found that perfect nails simply didn't exist. But if that be the case then what type of nails wins awards, you may ask?

This book is an answer to that question. You'll find the explanation here. You'll learn what the judges are looking for in a set of nails that is vying with others for the top place. I'll explain to you systems and strategies step by step to get you ready for the competitions. Those secret tips and tricks will also help you become a better nail technician if followed on a daily basis.

If you are a nail technician who would like to learn the trade or hone skills; or who has never entered a competition before and wants to know how and what to do; or who did poorly in a competition and would like to learn how to do better; then this the book for you. Here you'll find what it takes to become the winner and what others do to reach that top place.

If you're not sure you want to compete, don't worry. You may change your mind after reading this book. While I've gone into the technicalities of nail styling offering ample tips, I've also covered the necessary marketing aspect that you need to learn as a winner who also owns a business.

I've divided this book into three parts to dig deep into every aspect of nail styling and competitions, giving you as much information as possible. Part I (Getting ready for competitions) will teach you how to prepare yourself, what is important and what steps and actions must be taken if you want to do well on the big day. Part II (Competition day) tells you what to do and what to avoid on the D-Day. You'll also find here a products checklist and some important aspects of the competition that you and your model should bear in mind. Part III (After the competition) is about getting feedback, learning from your experience and making the most of it for your business using important marketing strategies writing PR copy to get your name out there.

This is your finest hour! An exciting venture is waiting for you!

WHY ENTER COMPETITIONS?

There are many reasons why you should enter a competition.

Let me ask you a question before we go any further. There are two hairdressers who've set up shop at the same time. One has never done any additional training, never been to any show, never competed courses while the other constantly learns, writes articles for magazines, does shows, takes part in competitions and sets standards. Whom would you chose to have your hair done by? The answer is simple, isn't it?

In the nail industry, too, customers prefer dynamic technicians because the industry is growing fast and fashions are changing all the time. What was popular two or even a year ago, may not be so any more. Trends, fashions, designs, techniques, shapes (in the nail industry) keep changing. One aspect, however, remains constant – that it's increasingly becoming tough to stay in business what with the growing number of nail stylist and also pseudo-stylists jostling for space. And if you don't do something to be in the reckoning, you're in trouble.

Nail competition is a game, so is the whole nail industry only rules are different. To be on top you must become a top player. You must deliver what others don't. You must be able to attract new customers and keep the regular ones in your fold by providing better and better services to them. It means you must become the nail technician that every client wants to go to and who has earned a reputation in the industry. Imagine a short street where five salons are located shoulder to shoulder. Only one of them has nail technicians who routinely take part in competitions. It's also the most expensive one. No prizes for guessing which salon is the busiest – the one that has award-winning technicians. Joining nail competitions is the key to your success.

You can build your reputation, position yourself in business and stand out from your competition by participating in contests. It makes you visible and may open the door for other opportunities that you think don't exist.

Every time you enter a competition, you grow. You become a better nail technician and better person. Despite fears and anxieties you do it anyway! Preparing for and taking part in a competition require a lot of discipline, determination, sacrifice, drive and passion. Everybody can enter competitions, but only a few actually do it. Why? Because it's a hard job and not everyone is willing to work hard and leave their comfort zone. You must become the person that does whatever it takes — no matter how hard it is — to shine through contests. When you do that you grow, so does your business and career.

Entering competitions gives you the opportunity to match your skills against others'. Most importantly, it's a test of how well you can handle your fears, doubts, and time! You must learn how to control your anxiety and emotions as well as focus on what is important and why you are there. These factors are your real competitors. So be prepared to give hundred per cent to win them all.

In fact, competitions teach you many things, but the most important of them are, being consistent, disciplined and determined despite stresses and fears. They also teach you that whether you're on the podium or not, you must always respect others as they worked as hard as you did.

Remember that even though winning is good, extremely satisfying and a goal at some point in your career, it's important to find out what it makes you, what you learn from this, and how all this can help your business and career.

One of my favourite quotes says:

> **"It's not who you are that holds you back. It's who you think you're not."**

You CAN do more than you think. Use this opportunity given by the nail industry to you to do things better, set standards and be a real winner.

PART I

GETTING READY FOR THE COMPETITION

SUCCESS PILLARS

Have you ever wondered why one person keeps winning competition after competition, or at least is placed second or third, while the others never make it to the podium? There's no doubt that she/he must have undergone a lot of training and is very talented and skilled. But is that all?

How is it possible that others, who're also very talented, never figure among the top three? Shouldn't they be winning too?

Experience tells me that entering contests any number of times doesn't ensure you success. You can enter one for the first time ever and win, or you can try many times with poor results or no results at all. Of nearly 20 championships that I have done, I've lost the top place only in two categories, either winning the rest or being on the podium leaving behind the others, more experienced competitors. How was this possible?

Nail championship is a game that involves not only your skills and abilities, but also your mindset and physical condition or general well-being. To be the winner you must be a fully packaged player your skills, mind and body must work in perfect harmony. Only then will you have a chance to win this game.

These three components — **skills, mind and body** — also require additional elements, which this book is all about, and they'll be covered in later chapters. For now, let's focus on these three pillars.

I. SKILLS

I'm sure you must have heard a tiny voice in your head saying, "I'm not as good as they are". You're not alone here; I've heard it before, too. Let's make it clear before we go any further no one is born with a brush and a file in their hand. Every single nail champion out there has worked really hard to get where they are now. Creating a stunning set of competition-standard nails requires great skills and abilities, and the only way to learn and develop your skills is through training and regular practice. Everyone is a potential champion, but very few are willing to do what it takes to become one. The good news here is that if you're motivated, focused, determined and have already acquired some skills, you are making your way to the podium.

Human being is a phenomenal creature. We are able to learn absolutely everything – from basic things like walking, writing or speaking to driving big buses, climbing mountains, or building high-rises. Creating competition-standard nails requires skills that you can learn. You must be shown and explained how to do that; then practise, practise and practise. Why do we have to keep practising? Because practice makes you... no, not perfect but <u>consistent!</u> This is the key to success in contests.

Before I ventured to do my first P&W competition, my educator had told me that I was rubbish there and that I should focus on nail art instead. She was right, as I wasn't great in many aspects and my smile lines looked like a sea wave. But I was determined to learn it, and I did learn. I believed that if others could do that, I could too.

Don't let your doubts control you and your actions. Just because something isn't great at the beginning doesn't mean it'll never be. You can learn whatever you want. It takes only your decision and commitment to do that; and when you actually do that, results and skills follow.

II. MINDSET

It's time to build a positive mindset, which is as important as sharpening your skills.

I'm pretty sure that before you register for a competition you will do a lot of thinking, talk to yourself and even wonder – am I really ready? Emotions of fear and excitement are absolutely normal. Most of us faced them before.

Despite those butterflies in your stomach, you take a bold step and register your name. Then you start training and practising like crazy, yielding mixed results. Often you wouldn't get the set of nails that you wanted so badly. Frustration creeps in and you start doubting your own abilities and regret having taken the big leap forward. Your subconscious mind tells you to stick to safer grounds of routine business and keep away from training and competitions. You're at a critical juncture, but **YOU'LL HAVE TO PRESS AHEAD** with your decision to participate in the contest. Tell that tiny voice in your head to shut up! Tell yourself that everything is just fine, and focus on what you're going to gain from the contest – a whole new experience. At the end of the day that's what really matters and that's what keeps you going.

If you're still not feeling ready to do the competitions, then let me tell you a story. Couple of years ago I had several students on my gel foundation course. Even though they were just beginners, I saw a great possibility in them and suggested that three of them enter a competition. They had been doing nails for only six weeks! That included their four-week-long course and a two-week period prior to the competition. They entered in the student category where they'd be competing with their peers who had been doing nails for at least six months. Of my girls, one came eighth out of the twenty-three contestants, another ended up third and yet another walked away with the entire category! Everything is possible.

I know it's easier said than done but you must find your **WHY** why you're doing it and why it is important to you. That's what will keep you motivated. Do you remember my educator telling me not to do P&W and stick to nail art instead? Yet I was determined not only to learn, but also to prove her wrong! I wanted to show her that everything was possible. When I was on the competition floor that day, I was scared to death; but I held on to my WHY for dear life. I knew that if I got a place I'd be living proof of making possible the seemingly impossible, and would live to tell that to my students.

Find your WHY, focus your full energy and thoughts on it, give your all to the competition, and watch what happens.

III. WELL-BEING

The third component, as important as the previous two, is your physical condition well-being.

On the big day you need your skills, mind and body to work in perfect harmony. That's why you'll have to make sure your health and well-being is in top condition. Trying to do a competition set with a runny nose would be very annoying. You need to stay healthy to stay focused; so you should look after yourself and avoid germs as much as possible.

Tiredness is your enemy. It slows you down, making it hard to concentrate on the competition. It's vital to have a good night's sleep before the big day. I, however, sometimes found that I was not affected much by the lack of sleep thanks to the adrenaline rush. I'd feel great and be on high alert during the competition, but would be drained of energy at the end of it. You might be thinking a surge of adrenaline on the D-Day would compensate you for staying up late the night before. No, it wouldn't help as most of the time you'd be doing two categories in one day, and you need high energy levels to last one full day.

It's perfectly all right to get nervous that day but never let your nerves take over. The moment it happens game's over! You must learn to control your nerves and play it cool. If meditation, or talking to someone, or treating yourself to a piece of cake makes you calm – go for it. In fact go for anything that helps you, as long as it's legal and appropriate.

As we can take care of our mind and body, there is, however, one thing that we can't do much about – ladies you know what

I'm talking about. If the big day happens to coincide with "THAT" day, make sure you've got your painkillers with you, just in case you need them. Every single factor matters, and if you can't concentrate on the competition hundred per cent you can't give hundred per cent.

Last but not least, you must be prepared to deal with emergencies calmly. Days of great preparation can be ruined in any moment. Things like funeral, illness of someone close to you, a sudden accident or even an insignificant argument may affect you a lot, and probably will. You can't control these things so take an appropriate decision on joining or leaving the contest in consultation with your family and friends. If no support is forthcoming from your family then you should bank on like-minded people for advice. This is crucial for you to be able to stick to what you've decided.

SETTING GOALS

It's the most important thing to do irrespective of whether it's your first or just another competition that you're taking part in. You must set a goal, or goals, for yourself to stay motivated throughout.

This must-do exercise will help you stay focused on the contest despite the little voice in your head discouraging you from joining the fray. The goals you've set will keep reminding you what really matters and why you should be doing what you're doing.

I, however, want you to keep in mind that goals aren't enough; they must be realistic too. If this is your first competition then you should aim to finish on time and to be in the top ten. There may be a little flutter in your stomach, but that shouldn't deter you from giving hundred per cent provided your targets are realistic. These are only suggestions and it is for you to take the right step. If you've already had the experience then you should aim for the podium, or do better this time round, or get more publicity and PR for yourself and your business. Again – be realistic. I always say, "Dream big, but set goals that you're capable of achieving; and feel good about them."

If you don't fix your targets right before the event it'll be as good as letting the competition slip through your fingers. Simply put, you will have no motivation and reason to be there. If these two elements are missing then contests aren't important to you, and if they aren't important, why do them at all?

Let me share with you how I set my goals not only before competitions, but also in my business and personal life. If you've never done anything like this before then it's going to be an eye-opener for you. It definitely was for me at one point in time! Here's an example of how goals are set, which I've learnt from T. HarvEker at one of his seminars.

1. **Step—Clarity**—What do you want?

   You have to very clear here the clearer the better. Decide what you want to do/achieve/get.

2. **Step**—**Why**—Why do you want it?

   What's it going to change/give/bring that makes you feel good when that happens?

3. **Step**—**Why not**—Why don't you have it yet?

   What's the reason? Maybe not enough training last time, or lack of good coach, nerves?

4. **Step**—**Strategy**—Your step-by-step HOW action plan.

   What do you have to do step by step to reach your goal? For example—follow this book :)

5. **Step**—**First action**—What can you do NOW or by this time tomorrow?

   Take action. Take a first, simple step that you can easily do, e.g., search for training.

6. **Step—Decide**—Make a commitment that you'll do it, no matter what!

    Your subconscious mind will try to trick you into believing that it's not doable, so a strong resolution is essential.

7. **Step—Reward**—Prize yourself.

    Once you've accomplished a task, give yourself a reward to remain highly motivated.

8. **Step—Accountability**—Have someone check on you.

    Find a coach, friend, or colleague, to whom you'll be accountable. Let him/her check your results and push you hard to better them.

This is the strategy I use. You may use a different one of course, but the point is: set the goal and achieve it. Start with something small and very easily achievable. You want to see and make sure that this system works. It does!

Stay focused, stay motivated and you'll do and get what you want.

FINANCES

I believe that every nail technician should do the competition at least once, as this could be one of the best experiences in their career. Having said that, I know how expensive it may be and that acts as a formidable deterrent to many techs.

Let's face it. You've got a registration fee to pay. Then you'll have to foot the bill for travel, accommodation, and meals, for your model (or models) and yourself. Add to it the fee that you'll have to pay your model(s). It all may come up to the price of a nice holiday. So if you don't plan your finances carefully ahead, you may find yourself in a sticky situation.

Here's how I plan and save money for my competition expenses, and you could do the same too.

I've got an empty jar in the salon, where I put all my tips from my lovely clients and a percentage of my salary. It's up to you of course to decide how much you can afford to set aside from your salary. The amount may vary every month depending on your tips and the cut from your salary that you lay aside. I'm sure you could easily save at least £100 a month doing it in this way.

Now, wouldn't your clients like to receive better and more comprehensive service from a nail tech who's also a champion? Of course they would. Why not to put your jar on your nail desk? Write a note on it, "Future NAIL CHAMPION," or whatever you think grabs their curiosity. Believe me it works. They're more generous than you think they actually are, especially when they know your WHY and can see a benefit for themselves in charity,

To avoid higher costs of registration you may avail of the early bird offer. It's worth doing as it saves you money that you can use on something else, such as travel or accommodation. Most of the competitions offer early-bird registrations just make sure you don't miss one.

Do your bookings — flight, train or hotel — well in advance. They'll be cheaper than last-minute arrangements plus they'll guarantee that you do get a ticket or a room.

You can't afford to forget your stock. If you're an educator and are also related to a brand, or a future tie-up with one is a distinct possibility, ask them to sponsor you. That could cover the products on your table, or competition fee, or one whole category, or something else. It's always worth asking that as you can save some money in this way. It's a win-win situation for both the company and you. The company gets exposure and free advertisement while you get their products or other benefits for free.

Planning your finances well ahead may save you — as also your other half — a lot of headache and stress. It's always better to plan in advance, so don't wait and start today!

COMPETITION REGISTRATION

This is the moment you finally take a decision to enter a contest. Congratulations! If you've already taken this step or are planning to do it.

There are many competitions in the UK and much more all over the world. Every nail competition is different. Rules for registration are also different, so are the criteria for competition nails. It's better to check with the event organisers what their rules are.

- **How do you register?**

  Most of the competitions are doing this online, where you download the form, fill it in and send it back with all your credit/debit card details. It can also be done by post, but check it out before you do it.

- **When does the early bird registration start and end?**

  You want to save yourself some money, so make sure you get the information and act accordingly.

- **When is the official deadline?**

  Once you've decided to enter a competition, you don't want to miss the deadline. There's nothing worse than that! Don't wait until last minute. If by any chance you forget about sending in your name, it may be too late by the time you remember to do it.

- **What is your division?**

  To register yourself in the right division (newbie, professional, and masters/veterans) is your responsibility. If you're not sure about it, contact the organisers for advice. You may be disqualified if you register in the wrong place.

- **Which category?**

  This is also your responsibility. Make sure you tick all the categories you want to enter and pay for all of them.

You will receive the registration and payment confirmation. Don't forget to carry printouts of them as you show up on the big day. You may need to produce them.

COMPETITION RULES

Rule one – Always read the rules! Every competition is different and has different rules. The rules of a previous competition may not necessarily apply to a new one as general rules, floor judge rules, rules for nail categories, and nails and judging criteria keep changing.

It's very common that rules are being modified every year for the same competition and even for the same category! You have to be sure that you know them before the big day. The last thing you want is to have points deducted for having or not having something on your table, or for using a product which is prohibited. Every point counts! Don't waste it. Once a student of mine forgot to line up for the bin and she lost 0.5 point. These things happen, but are they worth risking a point? Absolutely not!

General rules will tell you how the competition will look like; what is allowed or prohibited; how much time you'll have for each category; what exactly is expected of you as far as nails are concerned; and how they're going to be marked.

Floor judges are responsible for checking that general rules are being observed. They also mark that your products are on your table; health and safety measures are in place; your model is present; time is being maintained and you haven't stopped working.

Rule two – Always follow the rules! Never try to cheat or argue with the organisers unless there's been a mistake in printing those rules. Read them thoroughly and then follow them. If, for example, oil is not allowed, don't try to use it or else you may have points deducted. You may even be disqualified for that.

Sometimes, you'll be given hints and tips for a specific category, which are really valuable. Take a little time to study all information given, as this is part of your preparation. Knowledge is always better than ignorance! Even if you've entered a competition before, never ever assume that you already know a thing or two. For what you knew in the past may not apply this year.

JUDGING CRITERIA

A score sheet is an incredibly valuable thing, as it shows you in black and white which areas you are good at and where you need to work. It also the way the winner is selected.

Most of the inexperienced competitors think that the set of winning nails is the one that looks fabulous. Initially I also believed in it, but finally a moment came when I realised that it's a game and points mattered, not looks. What appears perfect from a distance may not look so good close up. For convenience, a set of nails is judged after it has been "broken" into smaller segments with marks assigned to each. Those nails that look good are most likely to win, but that's not always the case. In reality, the winning set of nails is the one that has made the least number of mistakes and scored most.

PERFECT NAILS DON'T EXIST. CONSISTENT NAILS WIN!

Do you understand now why this is a game? The nail game is all about consistency. It's about creating technically the same style across ten nails, making very few mistakes and collecting as many points as possible. You need to play it smart!

Through my competition training courses for both individual and group students, I teach all the winning techniques that I've learnt while doing courses and gleaned from my own experience. I teach how to do a set of competition nails consistently and how to avoid major mistakes. You can find it in great detail on **www. elaloszczyk.co.uk**.

As I said before, each competition is different with dissimilar judging criteria. However, they have some common elements for the judges to consider no matter where the contest is being held UK, Russia, Germany, Poland or any other country.

I'm going to talk you about them all now and focus on what is required. I'll also point out the most common mistakes and give you some valuable tips.

I. SHAPE OF THE FREE EDGE/FORM

- The shape is your choice;
- most common form is either square or squoval;
- has to be consistent across all ten nails;
- free edge is straight from the lateral fold and parallel;
- top of the free edge must be even;
- must not flare out or taper in;

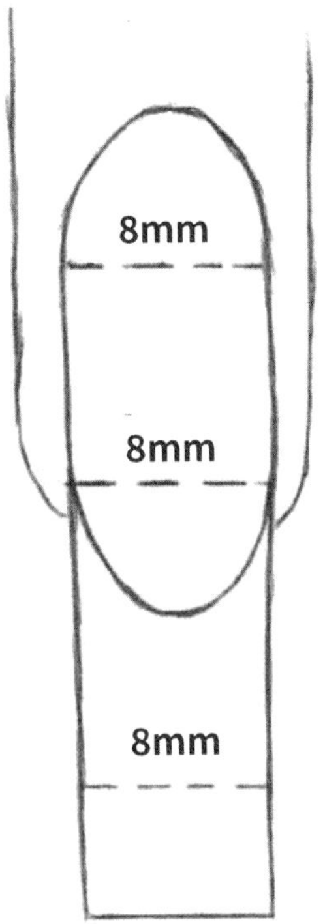

Most common mistake – top of the free edge isn't straight; nails are of different shapes; they taper in.

TIP!
Always keep viewing your work both from your side and your model's! Keep her hand straight to you and the file then turn around and view it from her side. Keep the free edge straight and even.

II. LENGTH

- Must be consistent and uniform across ten nails;
- in agreement with model's hands and fingers;
- may be measured – cuticle to centre of smile line, smile line to the free edge;
- measured from the cuticle area to free edge;
- consistent and matching nail to nail on the other hand (pinky to pinky, thumb to thumb etc.) and also matching the length on the same hand;
- the length varies from contest to contest, but the most common rule says – free edge mustn't be less than fifty per cent of the nail bed length and more than hundred per cent of the nail bed.

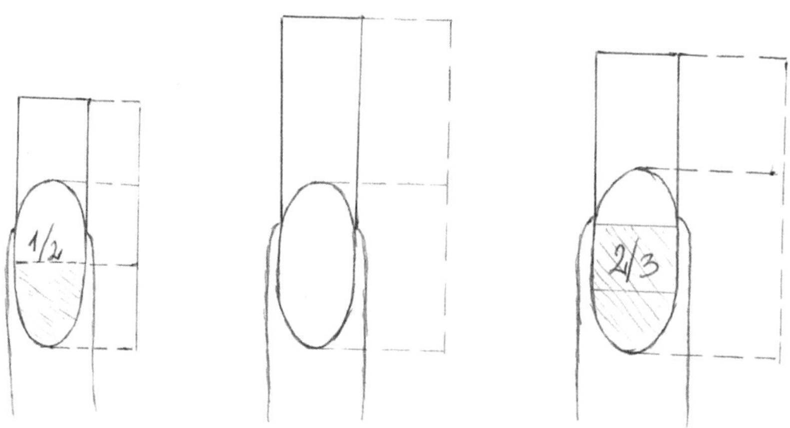

Most common mistake – nails don't match hand to hand.

PRACTICAL EXAMPLE:

Working fifty per cent: From cuticle to the deepest point of the smile line, when the nail bed each on the **middle finger** and the **thumb** is 20mm long, the length of the white extension for each finger would be 10mm from the deepest point of the smile line to the hairline, adding up to a total length of 30mm. The **ring** and **index fingers** each would then have a nail bed length of 19mm and a white extension of 9.5mm for a total length of 28.5mm. The length of the **small finger** nail bed would then be 18mm with a white extension of 9mm for a total length of 27mm.

Ring finger = Index finger in length.

Middle finger = Thumb in length.

The table below explains the world standard for nail lengths according to International Competition in Dusseldorf length 1:1 = 100% and 1:2 = 50%. You can use this table to work out for 60% or 80% lengths or anything else you want.

Length example 1:1 = 100%		
Nail bed	**White free edge**	**Total length**
10mm	10mm	20mm
11mm	11mm	22mm
12mm	12mm	24mm
13mm	13mm	26mm
14mm	14mm	28mm
15mm	15mm	30mm
16mm	16mm	32mm
17mm	17mm	34mm
18mm	18mm	36mm
19mm	19mm	38mm
20mm	20mm	40mm

Length example 1:2 = 50%		
Nail bed	**White free edge**	**Total length**
10mm	5mm	15mm
11mm	5,5mm	16,5mm
12mm	6mm	18mm
13mm	6,5mm	19,5mm
14mm	7mm	21mm
15mm	7,5mm	22,5mm
16mm	8mm	24mm
17mm	8,5mm	25,5mm
18mm	9mm	27mm
19mm	9,5mm	28,5mm
20mm	10mm	30mm

TIP!
Always keep checking the lengths nail to nail and then hand to hand. Do that before and after filing.

III. SIDELINES - SIDE AND FRONT VIEWS

- Extension aligns perfectly with the natural nail's lateral folds;
- from side view, sidelines should run parallel to one another;
- no excess material on lateral sides;
- no dents;
- from top view, the sidelines should not be wider than the natural nail's lateral sidelines or be filed away;
- the sidelines may be straight or very slightly tapered;
- sidelines from hairline view should be parallel.

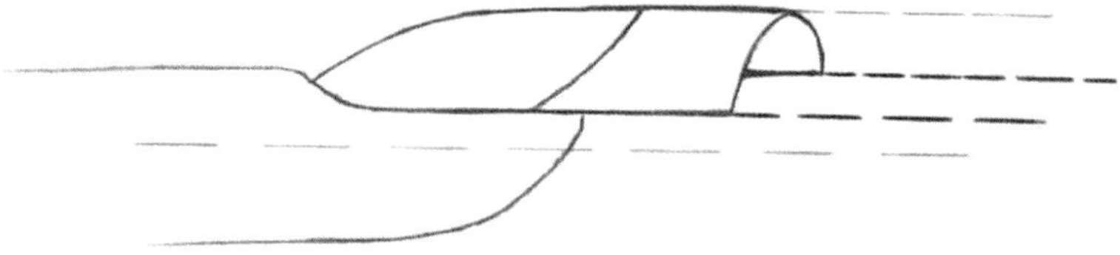

Most common mistake – sides are not parallel, dents present, or an excess of the product on lateral sides.

TIP!
In order to create perfect sidelines, start with the right way of tip application; follow it up with correct product application and filing technique. Make sure no product application is missing as it will create a hollow.

IV. ARCH/ APEX

- Consistent across all ten nails;
- placement depends on the competition style, rules and technician's choice;
- apex may be placed between 25% and 50% of the length from cuticle to hair line;
- two variants are possible – apex is close to cuticle and nail straight up to the free edge; or it's been moved closer to the centre of the nail and then free edge drops down slightly

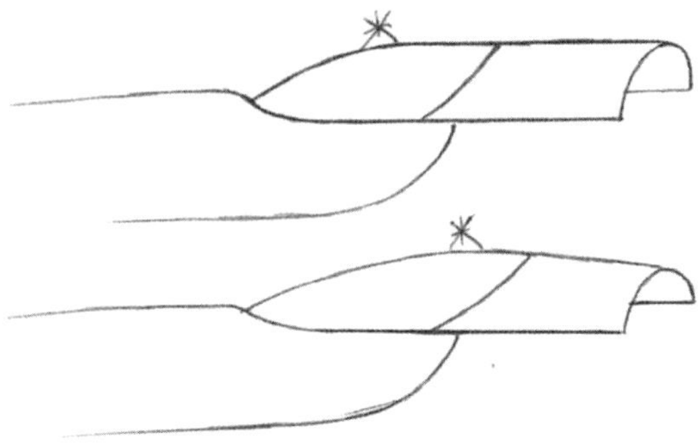

Most common mistake – inconsistent placement; placed too close to the cuticle area or too close to the free edge.

TIP!
Follow the cross method. Draw an imaginary cross on the entire length of the nail. The crossing point is your apex placement based on the natural nail length. It's 1/4 2/3 away from the cuticle area.

V. CONVEX

- Consistent across all ten nails;
- the exterior bevel is completely symmetric;
- no high or low points on the outer surface;
- nails must be evenly balanced and centred.

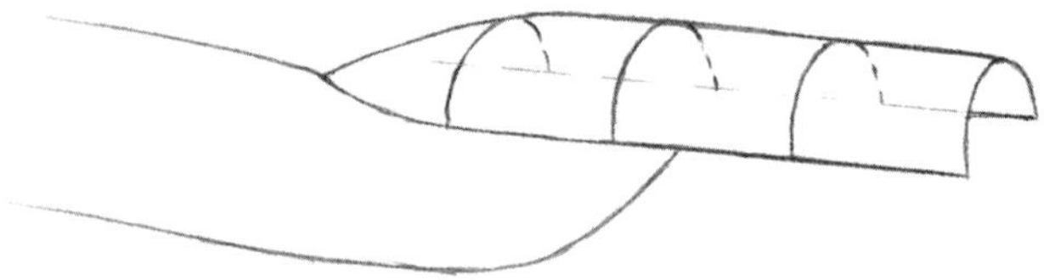

Most common mistake – inconsistent, centre point moved to the side.

TIP!
Pay attention to your filing technique and keep the centre in the centre of the nail. View it from model's side as well.

VI. CONCAVE

- Consistent across all ten nails;
- interior bevel is symmetric;
- no unevenness throughout the entire free edge;
- must have the same thickness across entire free edge;

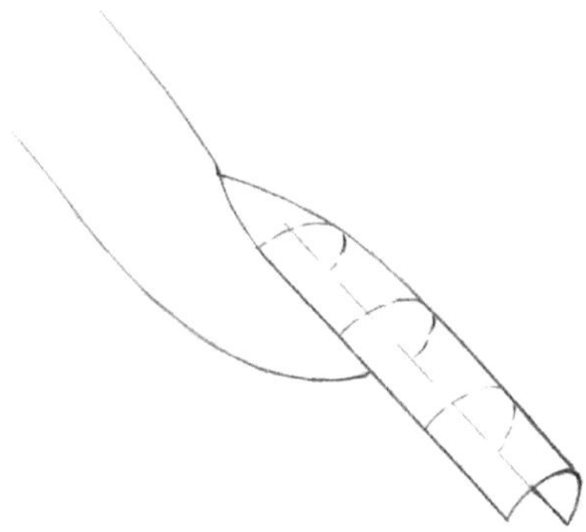

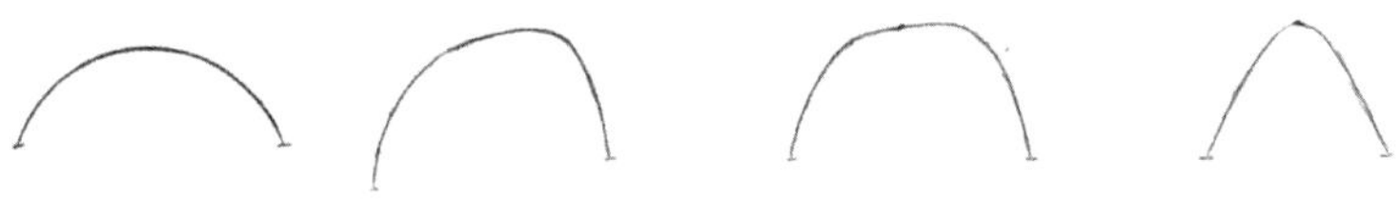

Most common mistake – sides too thin/thick compared to the top, or vice versa.

TIP!
The form application and even product distribution must be spot on. There should be no gaps between the form and natural free edge. Gaps make product too thick.

VII. C-CURVE

- Consistent across all ten nails;
- depth of curvature is between 40-50% of a circle, depending on the competition;
- must be symmetrical;
- the percentage of curvature is determined by model's natural nail shape and curvature.

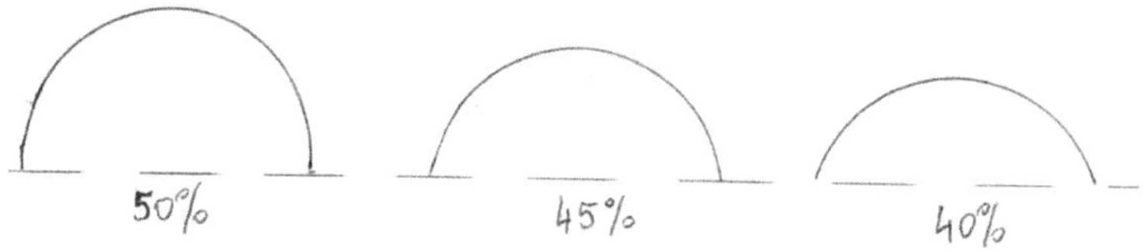

Most common mistake – improper, twisted form application; not pinching enough or over-pinching, no consistency.

> **TIP!**
> C-curve depends on form application and pinching technique; make sure you pinch at the right time so you won't squeeze the product creating hollows.

VIII. CUTICLE AREA

- No cuts or redness;
- product flash, perfectly blended around cuticle;
- no visible or palpable ledges;
- perfectly shiny close to the cuticle

Most common mistake – product is not flash or too much gap left between product and skin.

TIP!
Apply product very close and very thin around the cuticle, so filing is barely needed. You will make the nail around the cuticle shiny, but if there's no product in that area, the difference will be visible.

IX. HAIRLINE (FRONT OF THE FREE EDGE)

- The hairline should be as thin as a business card, or thinner;
- even and consistent across all ten nails;
- no thicker or thinner points around entire hairline;
- must be consistent across all ten nails.

Most common mistake – too thick or uneven.

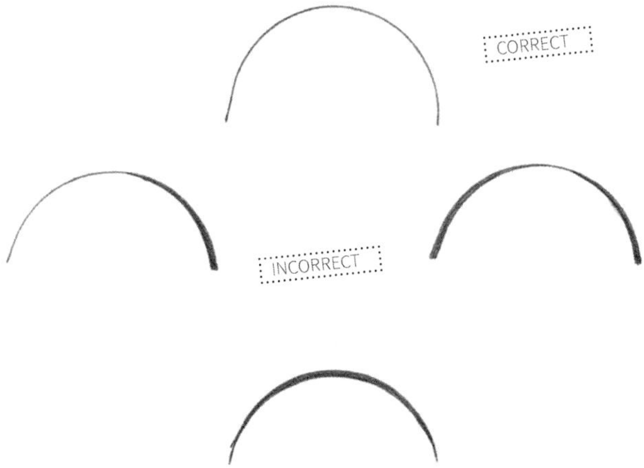

TIP!
Apply product thinly and evenly to avoid thickness and heavy filing.

X. SMILE LINE

- Consistent across all ten nails;
- crispy and sharp;
- corners of smile line are of the same height, crisp and even;
- consistent curvature;
- no shadowing or discolouration

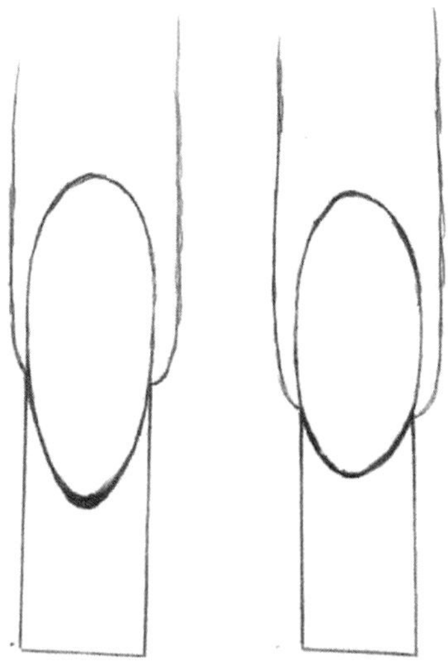

Most common mistake – inconsistent smile line, overfilled corners, or no corners at all, shadows.

TIP!
Product consistency is important here. Work corners right up to the side walls to be sure they don't disappear after filing.

XI. NAIL BED ELONGATION

- Consistent across all ten nails;
- perfectly blended around cuticle area and lateral side walls;
- visible from underneath – concave view;
- identical curvature of each nail;
- no bubbles or marble effect;
- lunula not covered.

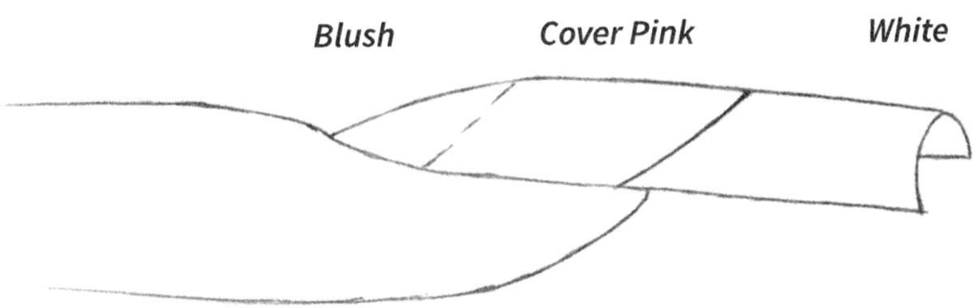

Most common mistake – product not blended well enough, inconsistent curvature.

TIP!
Use a mixture of cover pink and clear or blush for application to cuticle area. It will blend and look better.

XII. NAIL POLISH

- One hand (or two fingers if only one hand is being used) must be perfectly polished with two coats of cream nail polish;
- no colour on the skin;
- product application as close as possible to cuticle;
- perfect, consistent line at cuticle area;
- top of the free edge and lateral sides fully covered;
- no product under the free edge – concave view;
- no striping effect.

Most common mistake – product too far away from cuticle, uneven, on the skin and underneath.

TIP!
Use flat gel brush and acetone to clean cuticle line and skin.

XIII. TIP OR FORM FIT

- Tip must completely cover the groove-walls;
- extension must be perfectly straight to the nail and finger;
- mustn't drop or taper;
- no glue underneath;
- no visible tip on the nail bed;
- perfectly blended to the nail.

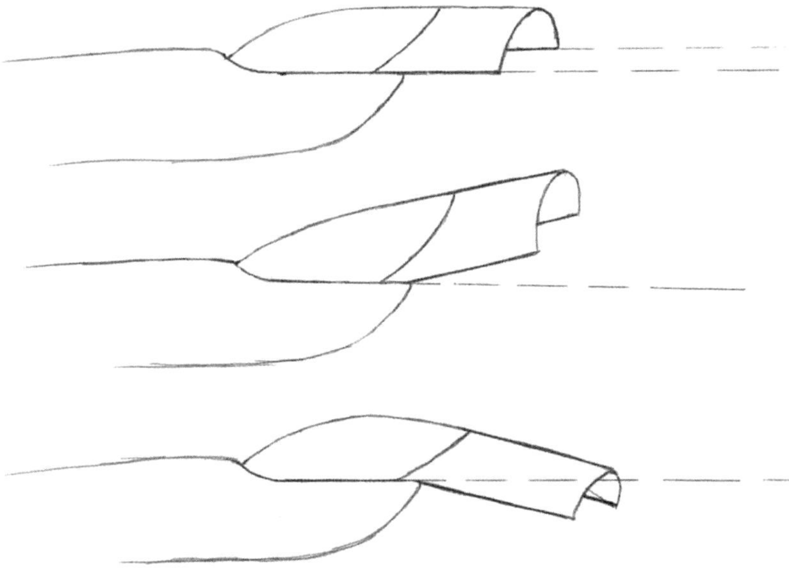

Most common mistake – tip too small, nails drop down, squint.

> **TIP!**
> Apply form straight to the finger not only to the nail; otherwise it will have a squint.

XIV. HIGH-SHINE FINISH

- High-gloss shine on unpolished nails;
- not visible after filing lines;
- entire nail, including edges, must be shiny;
- if allowed, top gel application must be even, smooth and shiny;

Most common mistake – edges or cuticle area visible, not shiny and not-fully-removed scratches.

> **TIP!**
> File nails using 180 grit file. It will be easy to eliminate scratches faster. Buff a lot! Use one buffer and shiner to one nail only.

XV. PRODUCT CONTROL

- No product on skin;
- no air bubbles and pits;
- free edge is white with no marble effect;
- nail bed elongation consistent in colour.

Most common mistake – white edge is marbled; air bubbles in pink/white.

> **TIP!**
> Correct mix ratio is crucial here. Don't pat product – stroke it.

XVI. OVERALL

- Full set is completely free from dust;
- no cuts or redness on skin and cuticle area;

- nails are smooth and glossy;
- **NAILS ARE CONSISTENT**

Most common mistake – dust underneath and dry cuticles.

> **TIP!**
> Use a bowl of water and cotton buds to clean under nails. (Unofficially speaking, ask your model to lick under nails and cuticles ;)).

These are the most common sections that judges mark. Your job is to make the minimum number of mistakes and score the most points! Become a “routine machine” and repeat every step on every nail exactly the same way.

CONSISTENCY is everything and it makes you win!

Check winning nails from previous competitions. Have a very close look and study them, as you may spot something that you haven’t seen before, and this may help you correct your mistakes.

The table below shows how judges score the nails. Remember that no common standards have yet been developed for nail competitions across the world. Each competition has its own standards, set by competitors themselves on the big day. Judges take a quick look first and then finalise the standards after seeing all nails.

Score guide – both hands	
10 Flawless	**5** Average
9 Almost flawless	**4** Below average
8 Very good	**3** Poor
7 Good	**2** Very poor
6 Above average	**1** Unacceptable

Score guide – one hand
5 Flawless
4 Very good
3 Average
2 Below average
1 Very poor

There are several occasions when you may have some **points deducted** for reasons that entirely depend on the type of the competition you're in, but the most common are:

- Not following the general or floor judges' rules;
- using prohibited products;
- broken or unfinished nails;
- using mobile phones;
- disturbing other competitors.

IDEAL MODEL

Finding an ideal model may be the hardest part of the game. She is extremely important, comprising almost fifty per cent of your success! Just imagine yourself working on someone who's got squint fingers, each nail has a different length and a very high natural apex and looks like a hook. It's going to be extremely hard to make a competition set of nails out of them. It will cost you a lot of stress and require great skills and experience. Go easy, spend a little more time looking for the best model that you can have.

I'll tell you what to focus on when looking for one, but first let's answer the burning question: Where are you going to find her?

Start with your clients. I'm sure you can think of a client whose nails stand out from those of the others. If such a one is hard to come by, look for one in your family, friends, their friends and so on. You may also check Facebook, Instagram, model agencies, and even advertise or just spread a word to that effect. It's not the easiest thing to do, yet so important and beneficial.

Here's what you'll be looking for regarding hands and nails:

- The WOW factor – you'll know exactly what that means once you find the right person;

- smooth and young skin;
- slim and straight fingers;
- healthy colour and good skin condition;
- long, oval nail beds – at least 1.5cm;
- nails without high apex;
- straight side walls (no funny-shaped nails);
- lateral walls not high;
- flexible fingers.

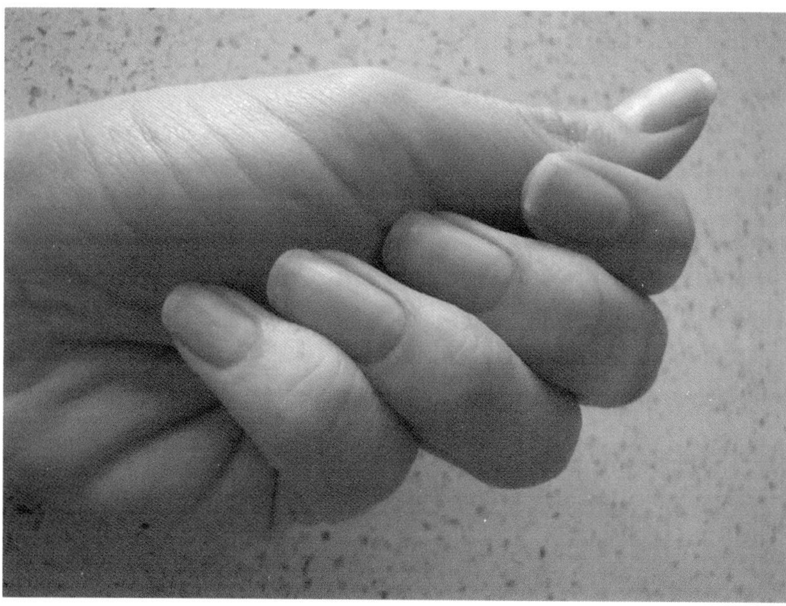

Let me give you now some tips on **how to create a portfolio of your models and how to take photos.**

1. Model's contact details: full name, phone number.

2. Take a photo of her face – it's good to know your model by face and not by her hands alone.

3. Take a close photo — top view — of her both hands placed flat.

4. Take a close photo of both thumbs placed flat.

5. Measure her nails, both hands. Do the left hand starting with pinky: LP, LR, LM, LI, and LT. Follow the same with her right hand.

6. Make a lot of notes, e.g. apex height, skin condition, scars, birth marks etc.

Print out those photos and keep them in one folder with all the details. You may be thinking that you don't have to do that as she's your client and you know her hands and all. But this is crucial. You must study and memorise every detail of your main model's hands and nails, so you don't have to think how to apply form etc.

You should be very happy when you come across such a person that ticks all the boxes, but that's not all. There's also another side to the ideal model and that is her personality. She must feel at one with your team. What I mean is, she must co-operate with you and be a genuine well-wisher urging you on to win. You should know that you can count on her and that she'll do whatever is necessary to bring you closer to win. She must be willing to lick those cuticles, if needed. She should stay calm all the time although you may become a bundle of nerves.

Life is unpredictable and sometimes throws a challenge at you. I had my share of it some years ago. On the competition day, my model grew nervous and her hands started sweating a lot. Sticking forms to her fingers was impossible. After several failed attempts to do so, I desperately tried to dry her hands with just anything — sanitiser spray, acetone, dehydrator — but nothing worked. Precious minutes ticked by. I thought I was finished! Finally, after ten minutes of cracking jokes to calm her down, and lots of acetone, I managed to dry her hands just enough to stick forms. I ended up third.

Another competition and another model. This time, ten minutes to end of the competition, I broke the corner of the index finger nail when buffing to a high shine. I panicked and didn't know what to do. My model was horrified. "Oh f.... what have you done! Do something, do something," she said. Somehow her reaction helped me gather myself. I had no time to remove the nail and do it all over again, so I quickly filed the top, applied form again and built the corner. The damage was slightly visible but the nail looked complete and that's what mattered. This time I ended up second.

You and your model must be prepared to deal with any kind of situation. Control damage in a creative way as this will have a great impact on the final results. NEVER give up! There's always a solution to a problem. Find it.

You'll need to spend a lot of time practising on her. You should practise on your clients too. You can also switch to metal C-curve sticks if your clients are unwilling to co-operate with you, but more about that later.

Your model should spend a lot of time with you. She must be flexible and willing to do that. She may track the time for you. Every competitor has their own way of doing it. My model tells me how much time is left. That helps me a lot. During a competition, the time is announced every half or one hour, so there's no problem for you. But I personally don't like that. I often ask my model to tell me the time after adding five minutes to it. So I'm always ahead of real time until the final 15 minutes. However, if I'm behind my time, she prods me to work faster and tells me the exact time left. That works fine for me.

The role of your model is not limited to letting you use her hands and nails. She is your co-competitor and both of you are fighting a common battle shoulder to shoulder. Nurture that relationship and treat your model well.

Before the competition begins, it'd be wise of you to keep one or two more models handy. Your main girl may not be able to accompany you for reasons beyond her control, as you set out to participate in a contest. Your backups save you a last-minute desperate search for a fresh model.

If you have no backup then you can very well hire someone to do it for you. Many people, especially those who travel very far to join a contest, are known to do that. Hiring one of the locals at the venue turns out to be cheaper since you don't need to worry about their travel or accommodation expenses. The flip side is that you're unlikely to get a chance to practise on her even once prior to the competition. She'll be an unknown quantity. You won't know her personality and nature. Will she motivate you to win the contest as your regular would have done? Will she keep track of the time for you? You don't know. If you want to go for such a model, make sure you have a good agreement with her to avoid nasty surprises.

Practising on your model is important and a must; however, don't work too hard on her nails and hands as these will have to be kept in top condition. There are several things that shouldn't be done close to the competition day.

Things you should NOT be doing on a model the day before the competition:

- DON'T remove cuticles as on the competition day you'll be filing faster and harder and that may cause her sensitive skin to bleed. There's also the risk that she may get some cuts in the process. It's going to cause a lot of pain, and points may be deducted for redness around cuticles. Do a full manicure a week in advance and then just soak the fingers a day before.
- DON'T give a paraffin wax treatment. Wax may leave too much oil on natural nails and skin, making it difficult for you to stick nail forms to the finger. As a result, product may not adhere to the nail. HOWEVER, your model should use a lot of moisturising cream every day (after washing her hands) and over the night to keep her finger skin soft and hydrated.
- DON'T practise on your model. Over-filing may create redness, make cuticle sensitive, and change the colour of natural nails.
- DON'T remove acrylic or gel. That should be done at least two days before the D-Day to make sure that nails and hands are in good condition. It will also give them a small break between all those applications and removals.

If you are serious about the competition and really want to increase your chances to win, make sure you'll do everything you can to find a model described above. Your skills bring only fifty per cent of success to the table. The other half depends on your model.

COMPETITION TRAINING

If you are serious about competition and you're going there to do well then you have to do competition training, especially if this is your first time, or you didn't get the results you wanted last time. I'll say it not once, but hundred times every single competitor must do this training.

Want to know why? Here's feedback from my student, who did a course with me and got results:

> *"After many years of attending competitions I finally decided to take the competition course with Ela. I kept coming up second or third so felt like I needed that extra guidance, which was exactly what Ela gave me. The training was on for a full day and was so in-depth that it gave me a better understanding of what the judges would be looking for in the shape of the nail as well as what competition nails were all about. It was definitely worth doing it since some months later I came first in three categories that I'd chosen to compete in! I highly recommend training with Ela who is so professional in her manner and very attentive to what you need to work at."*

***Ania Kesiak**, Nails for You*

That's what I teach my students and the results they have afterwards. The benefits of this training are endless (**www.elaloszczyk.co.uk**).

There's a huge difference between salon nails and competition nails. I'm sure you already can see it after reading the judging criteria chapter. As a competitor and judge, I'm often amazed by the fact that some people enter competitions without proper training. They get really surprised when it doesn't turn out as expected. It's time to face the reality – if you think that you can walk in and win competitions without proper training, then wake up. This just doesn't happen, unless you are super-talented and extremely skilled. The truth is, most of the champions out there worked really hard to get where they are now. They didn't get success overnight. It came through hard work and preparation which had started with competition training.

One of my favourite quotes says:

Fail to prepare, prepare to fail.

Preparation and training are your ticket to success. Every successful competitor has done it and, believe me, it never stops with one training course.

Why should you do several competition training courses with various coaches? No two technicians are same and no two techniques work the same way. We all are different and think differently. Two trainers using the same technique would teach you in as many different ways. They would tweak it separately to make it work for you. So learning from many educators gives you an opportunity to collect a whole range of techniques and then wisely select from it which one you want to use and when. That's the trade secret.

Let's dig deep into the subject and focus on its important aspects.

1. INDIVIDUAL OR GROUP TRAINING?

That depends on your learning preferences. What type of training will be more beneficial for you? Do you get better results under individual training *with all the attention riveted on you,* or you could get the same results from training in a group *without all that attention?* I went for individual training when I first took one and I strongly recommend it. I didn't know until then how competitions looked like or how nails should look like. I felt that I'd be better off doing a one-to-one course because it was my first training of this kind. Also, I wanted some personal tips and was hoping to learn a few tricks from my educator who taught me alone. Later I did more one-to-one and group training courses which were very helpful too. You could immensely benefit from group training if you knew what you're doing and what your goal was. Either training would be fine as long as you got one right before a competition that you're joining.

2. EDUCATOR

How to find one and what to look for in them? There are many educators out there offering various competition training courses. Here's a small guide to help you choose the right one who'll prepare you for the big day.

- His/her **experience as a competitor**. Whoever is going to teach you must have exposure to competitions otherwise you won't learn much about contests from that person. It is not necessary that you should be taught by a winner, but if they have a long experience of doing the competition circuit, it'll help you get there.
- His/her **experience as a coach, educator.** You should learn from someone who has a proven track record of not only teaching foundation classes, but also preparing students for competitions. That's what matters here. What can you expect from them? What will you learn? How is their experience going to benefit you? For answers to these queries have a look at the person's profile and achievements but, most importantly, get **student feedback.** It'll also be extremely beneficial for you if the coach is a judge too. Then he/she knows exactly what to pay attention to and how to get you closer to your goal.
- His/her **students' achievements, results**. You want to be sure that your investment is going to pay off. But to be honest, not every student will shine forth with great results as they depend on individual skills, experience, and tenacity of spending hours on practice. Those who follow the plan and do whatever it takes, succeed in life. Check student feedback, results, and achievements. Discuss with them the benefits they've had from the training. Remember that preparation for competitions not only increases your chances to reach the podium, but it also makes you a skilled nail technician who provides better and more consistent service. It will benefit you in all areas of business and career.

"I have recently been trained by this lovely lady, and I have to say she certainly knows what she is talking about; fantastic day and I learned loads. She is very patient and teaches in a way that you can understand."

***Sharon Dumper**, 10 Pampered Pinkies*

3. WHEN SHOULD YOU DO THIS TRAINING?

It depends on your skills and abilities. You can start about two months before the competition if you are a fast learner and can easily adopt new techniques. However, anything done well in advance is always more beneficial as it gives you plenty of time to get used to these new techniques and practise them a lot.

The longer you train the better you learn. But there's no golden rule. Even if you do your training a month before the competition, you could do well too. But then you won't have enough time to prepare and practise. This can cause a lot of strain and stress to you; so make sure you start training early enough to prepare well for the contest.

Also remember that if you want to take an individual training course, then plan and do it months in advance. This will help adjust your schedule with that of your educator. So don't forget to enrol in advance.

4. TRAINING IS AN INVESTMENT IN YOURSELF

Every time you take a course and learn something, you invest in yourself. It's probably the best investment as money spent on your personal growth affects the entire area of activity such as your business, service time and quality, clients etc. Always invest smart and never go for something just because it is cheap.

The cost of the training will depend on the expertise of your educator as described above, but mostly on the educator's experience and his/her students' results.

Individual training courses are always more expensive than the group variety. But if you find that training with a particular coach will help you learn something valuable that will help your career and business, go for it. Price shouldn't be an issue here. A pricey training never deterred me from going ahead and doing it when I knew that the educator could deliver something that justified the high price. For such training, I often had to travel abroad with my model in tow so I could practise on her what I'd learn. The expenditure went up so did the line on my career graph! For expensive courses you must carefully plan your expenses in advance. Everything is possible; you just have to plan it.

I encourage you to do competition courses and to learn from as many educators as you can. Make a list of coaches you want to train with and make it happen. This is what I do. I've got such a list and I plan in advance to be sure I can afford it.

P&W COMPETITION STYLES

What I like about P&W competition is that it's flexible. You have the option to choose the system you want to work with – acrylic or gel. Always pick the one you're comfortable with and can get better results with. I've trained in both systems and do both when working with my clients. P&W acrylic sculpt is my forte and I love doing it although I've done tips and gel and won awards in those categories with them. But acrylic sculpt will always be my first choice.

While working in a salon, you must find out which system you feel more comfortable with. Stick to it and develop your skills further in this area. Concentrate on that with full energy results will follow.

P&W competition allows you to decide in which category you'd like to compete. Your choice could be:

- sculpting or tip and overlay;
- competition standard or salon standard (softer criteria).

The choice is yours. You can do one or all of them if the competition time schedule allows.

Other P&W variants are:

- you can do classic "french";
- use a cover pink to extend the nail beds.

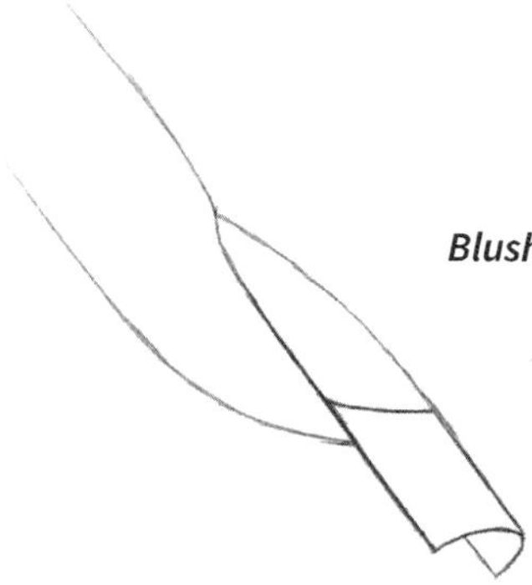

- Moons may or may not be required. If required (natural nail's lunula must be covered or created with soft white powder), make sure you work with dry and very small beads;
- apex placement – two variants are possible;

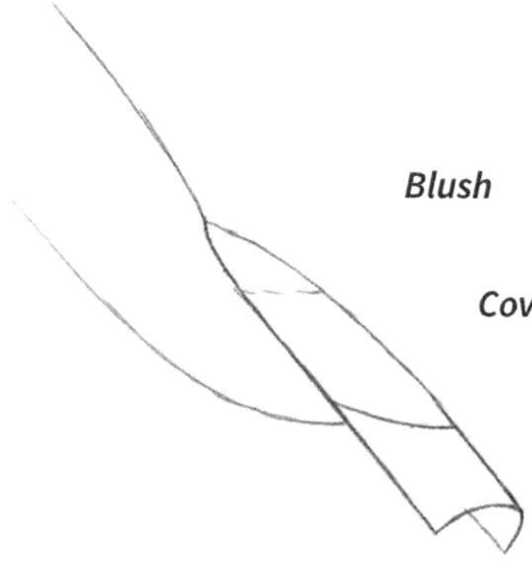

- curvature of smile line – either a soft ended V, or a U shape;
- some competitions allow you to use electric drills and oil;
- white tips are prohibited, only natural or clear are allowed. Do one of them with a very deep C-curve.

One of the most visible differences in competition styles is the length of the nail bed elongation and free edge. Styles and standards vary from contest to contest, country to county, For example, the Russian standard may be different from the German or there'd be little similarity between the Polish or German styles etc. In the UK, too, competitions have dissimilar rules and standards. So read the rules carefully before you proceed.

PRACTICE SCHEDULE

You must practise hard to make the most of your training and there are no two ways about it. Competitions require you to spend a lot of time on getting ready. You also need courage and determination, and should be ready to sacrifice pleasure for business. It's a hard job but very rewarding.

Fortunately, there is a system how to practise in a smart way to get the best results. I'm going to share it with you now.

First of all, follow the guidelines given in this book. Train your hands and mind to make a habit of creating winning sets of nails. "We are what we repeatedly do," Aristotle says. What does it mean?

You require time and patience to do the same thing over and over again and only then can you create a habit of making winning nails consistently. Psychologist Jeremy Dean in his book *Making Habits, Breaking Habits: "Why We Do Things, Why We Don't, and How to Make Any Change Stick say that it takes about 21 days to make a small and simple habit."*. However, if it's more complex than drinking a glass of water in the morning, more time is needed.

What has this got to do with our training? You'll have to practise hard for at least 21 days and make it a habit if you want to implement all of the techniques that you've learnt on your competition training. I can imagine you saying, "But I don't have time for that!" Bear with me, don't give up just because it's hard.

Practising on a model (your main model) is the best way to start. But after 21 days of doing a model, you'd hardly be left with any natural nails to work on. Therefore, you should also use the C-curve sticks for the purpose. Pick up one; any size you like, and put sculpting form on it as if it's a model, making sure that the form is not fully on the stick and that it creates a free edge. Practise product application every day and do at least one nail a day; this trains your hands and brain in the process. A habit is born.

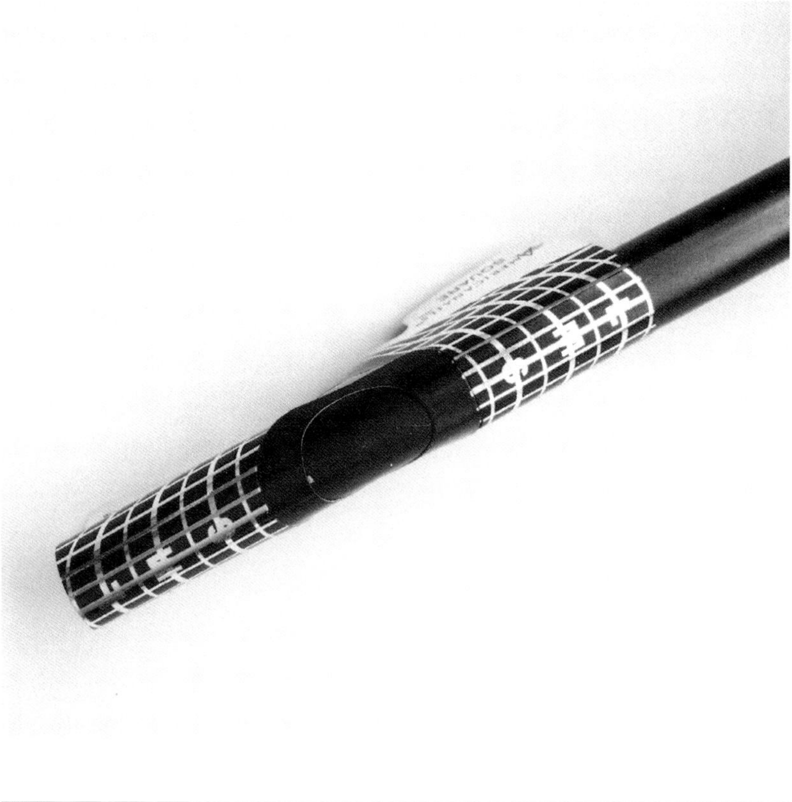

Now practise on models, the type of training you mostly want to do, and it helps you gain valuable experience. You'll have to devote 2.5 hours a day to doing a set (see contest rules for time allotted to your chosen category), the exercise also includes other related tasks, such as making pre-training preparations and removal or shortening of nails after. I personally recommend that you leave the nails untouched until next training and that minimises the risk of damage. One of my coaches advised me to practise on a model for three days in row for X period of time. World-class nail guru Tom Holcomb, who died in October 2011, however, said he always started training two weeks before a competition, working for four hours a day on the same model. I train months in advance at least once a week on a model and every day on sticks. Two weeks to the competition, I increase training on model up to three times a week.

Practising daily on models would help you make a habit of it pretty fast. Set the time apart, organise your models and follow a system that works well for you.

Let's recap quickly – practise for at least 21 days in a row in order to create a habit. Practise full sets on models and use C-curve sticks every day doing at least one "nail". Chose the system which works for you and stick to that.

Remember that doing a couple of full sets just before the competition won't be enough. Start your preparations months in advance as it's safe to be in a contest with plenty of practice. Do everything you can to get results that sparkle.

Moving on to **timing your practice**. Competitors have their own systems of practice. I'll share mine with you, which can be followed or tweaked to convenience. Do what works for you.

I divide my 2.5-hour-long practice session into sections. I always try to follow this system and stick to my timing. But if I spend a little more time in the first section I try to make up for it in the second by speeding up work. During training, you may sometimes finish before time but don't waste it doing nothing. Use it to fine-tune your work – buff those nails so that they look their best, make sure cuticles are nice and soft and there's no dust or polish on the skin etc. In short, use it to make the most of your performance.

Segments of a CLASSIC P&W set	Time schedule for both hands
Preparation includes pushing back cuticle, filing free edge, removing shine and dust, applying dehydrator and primer	5min
Form and product application includes form prep and application, white and pink product application and pinching C-curve	80min
Filing + buffing + shining	45min
Nail polish	15min
Finishing involves cleaning the skin from any nail polish, dust and double checking whole set	5min

When you use cover pink to elongate nail beds you may find that product application takes more time. If that's the case, speed up filing or polishing to make up for lost time. In competitions, cover pink doesn't come with extra time.

Segments of P&W set with cover pink	Time schedule for both hands
Preparation includes pushing back cuticle, filing free edge, removing shine and dust, applying dehydrator and primer	5min
Form and product application includes form prep and application, white and pink product application and pinching C-curve	90min
Filing + buffing + shining	35–40min
Nail polish	10–15min
Finishing involves cleaning the skin from any nail polish, dust and double-checking whole set	5min

During practice, always finish the whole set of nails on time. It is very important to do so. Imagine you're in a contest so complete each set and don't leave a session before it is over. It pays to mimic the big day by setting your table properly, starting your work with some gravitas and finishing the whole set of nails on time. Also, teach you model how she could be helpful on the D-Day.

Ideally, the timing of your practice session should match that of the competition that you're aiming to join. For example, if it's scheduled to start at 8 a.m. on a particular day, you should begin your practice that early. This would enable you to get used to the big day schedule. If you're a late riser it'll get you habituated to beginning your day early in the morning.

Make the most of every training session, keep pushing yourself to do better. You really have a lot to gain.

Once again remember that the winning set of nail is the one with the fewest mistakes. Play this game smartly and earn as many points as you can.

PART II

COMPETITION DAY

TOOLS AND PRODUCTS

There are no magic products which will create a great set of nails for you. But you can have the best the one you like most and get very good results from. What works best for you may not suite someone else, so an objective evaluation of nail tech products would be pointless. On the competition day, use the products that you've practised with and never make any last-minute changes as your hands are used to a particular gel or acrylic. Don't forget that your white should be pure white, not greyish; transparent pink shouldn't be too dark and cover pink must blend easily and match the model's skin tone. If your products don't tick all the boxes, do some research and come up with the right ones. Get used to them months before the competition.

I personally like medium – fast setting acrylics and thin gels. They work perfectly with my strategy. When I do classic P&W acrylic set, I sculpt one whole nail (I always start with the little finger), next I apply form on the second finger, and then I go back to my pinky as it is ready to be pinched and so on. When doing gels, I use thin clear gel because it levels much faster and there's less work and filing to do. I'm not a fan of fast setting acrylics as they don't give enough time to work on the smile line and the length.

I'm sure you already know which products you like better – faster or slower setting, runny or builder gels. However, familiarity with products doesn't always help. They may behave in a funny way as temperatures fluctuate, forcing a change in the way you normally work. You can't predict temperatures for the competition day or the venue. A huge hall hosting the contest probably will be colder than your salon or room. When temperature drops acrylic sets slower and gel thickens. In the event of such a possibility, a thermos of hot water and a bowl should also accompany you to the competition. If the low temperature of the venue makes your acrylic set slower then pour the liquid into your dappen dish and put it in the hot water bowl. The liquid will be back to normal soon. You can give the same treatment to your gel.

On the other hand, higher temperatures make acrylic set faster and the gel becomes runny. In this case you use ice-cold water to set things right. It's the easiest and quickies way to solve your temperature problems at competitions and you can try this in your salon too.

Talking about products, if you plan to use cover pink and soft white you need to remember a thing or two about them. Cover pink for nail bed elongations should match your model's skin tone and create naturally looking colour. Avoid those candy pink or brownish covers, unless they match your model, as they're hard to blend with natural nails. The soft white acrylic will be used to sculpt the moons, but many competitions don't need them. If you don't have soft white prepare it by mixing 1 part normal white with 3 parts clear. However, the particular products you use may work best at a different proportion so try various combinations to find it.

SPECIAL TOOLS I USE AND RECOMMEND

- **Pinching clamps**

  I like them better than manual, metal tweezers, as they're easy to use and don't waste my time. Just place them on, secure, and you're ready to move on to the next nail. They're very light and hold the nail easily in a tight grip. You don't risk your model squinting or loosening them. They can be plastic or metal.

- **Metal file**

  This is very useful for filing sides of the nails. You'll be able to reach those narrow sides much easier with this than with an ordinary file. You could also use a manicure file. It's not, however, as strong as the metal one and may bend easily.

- **C-curve sticks**

  I use them for two things:

  To correct my C-curve and make sure it's uniform; and to use it as a file. I cut a piece off a 150 grit file and glue it to the top of the stick. This is how I make a round file, and use it to file the concave of the nails if necessary. It comes in very handy in competitions where the use of e-file is prohibited. Those who don't use an e-file can have a look at it.

- **Metal form**

  It helps in sculpting a set of nails and takes care of the shape, C-curve, concave, and parallel sides. It also cuts the pinching time to a minimum.

- **Well-less tips with very deep C-curves**

  They eliminate blending to a minimum and allow you to get really deep C-curves through further pinching.

- **Cotton buds**

  Many people use a manicure bowl and water to clean all dust from the nails. I personally like using cotton buds soaked in water to do it. I find it better and more precise. Some also use compressed air to get rid of dust, which also gets blown around and eventually settles on the model's polished hand.

- **E-file**

  I use it where it's allowed. There's no faster way to blend tips, prep nails, or gently file the cuticle areas without actually touching and irritating them. It's a great time-saver.

PRODUCTS CHECKLIST

As I know how stressful competitions can be, I've made a products checklist so you won't forget anything important. Add or remove any items if required, but having too many products on the checklist is better than too few showing up on it.

If you forget to take something, don't panic. You can always buy it, if the competition doubles as a trade show, or borrow from someone. Never focus on a problem, but on finding the solution.

The check list below shows you all the products you need to take with you. You may pack gels or acrylics if the category you're contesting in requires it.

Gel products:	Acrylic products:	Other liquids:
• base gel	• clear powder	• dehydrator
• top gel	• soft white	• primer
• clear gel	• mega white	• acetone
• cover pink	• transparent pink	• alcohol
• transparent pink	• cover pink	• water
• white	• liquid	• oil – if allowed
		• hand lotion
		• red nail polish

Files and buffers: • manicure file • metal file • 180 grit files • 150 grit files • 100 grit files • white bloc buffers • 180/100 grit buffers • 220/280 grit buffers • 400/6000 shiners	**Brushes:** • acrylic brush • gel brush • manicure brush	**Other tools:** • 2 dappen dishes • nail forms • nail tips • tip cutter • glue • cuticle pusher • cuticle nipper • scissors • metal pinching tool • plastic pinching clips • C-curve sticks • orange wood sticks
Electrical equipment: • table lamp • bulbs • UV lamp • LED lamp • electric drill • drill bits • dust collector • extension lead	**Other necessities:** • cotton buds • nail wipes • paper towel • table towel • brush wipes	**Health and safety products:** • hand sanitizer • tool disinfectant • disinfectant jar • client consultation form • safety glasses • gloves • metal bin • bin linen

Also, some competitions prohibit participants from using certain products or even displaying them on their tables. Refer to the competition rules for more information.

PROHIBITED PRODUCTS:

- oil;
- ridge filler;
- base or top coat;
- glue (sculpting category);
- gel top coat (acrylic category).

THE BIG DAY

Finally it's arrived, putting an end to your hard preparations and long anxious wait. You're probably going to be stressed, nervous, and even panicky as you approach the venue. Your body language reflects the state of your mind which is so poorly coping with a range of emotions. That's absolutely normal!

When I entered my first competition, I couldn't sleep the night before, couldn't eat, and felt like someone was squeezing and twisting my stomach. Waiting for the results was even worse. I still go through these feelings every time I compete. In fact, the moment you stop feeling all that on the competition day, you stop caring about your career and life. Whenever you feel that way about competitions or yourself as a nail technician/educator – change your profession. You'd never again find it exciting and it becomes a routine job rather than a passion.

You need to know several important things about the big day — some do's and don'ts — and I have divided them into the following two segments:

I. YOU

- **Get up early and have a good breakfast and something to drink**. I know it is very hard, but you must do that as you're going to need a lot of energy. If you're competing in more than one category a day, you may have no time to eat. Don't skip breakfast and always take some food, or at least some chocolate bars, with you to eat later in the day. Don't forget about the needs of your model.
- **Don't drink too much beverage** as there's no time for restroom brakes. This is going to be one of those long days. Make sure you're able to control your body's natural needs without drinking too much. Let me remind you once again that your focus should be on doing the best you can with nails, not on anything else.
- **Wear your uniform or promotional T-shirt, apron, or dress.** Some competitions require you to wear uniform while others are mum on the issue. But you should look professional all the time. Make sure you present yourself well, as photos for magazines will be taken any time. The occasion also provides a chance to promote the brand that has sponsored you. Dress properly, have your make-up and nails done, and hair tied back.
- **Arrive at the competition early** to avoid a queue at the entrance. You're already stressed and nervous so the sight of a sea of people jostling at the entrance won't soothe your nervous. Early birds will get the best of seats and this is the last thing you want. Arrive earlier. You may have to wait couple of minutes to get inside, but it'll save a lot of unwanted stress.

- **Check in at the registration desk to get a number**. This is your responsibility. Again, the rules vary from event to event, but it's usually tagged to your model's hand and your T-shirt or uniform. This is your unique number and the judges will mark your model with that. They don't know names.
- **Choose a good seat away from drafts and visitors.** A flow of air or draught may cause bubbles in your products so stay away from those seats if you can help it. Choose a place away from the aisle to avoid getting distracted by onlookers. However, if you feel that crowds motivate you, take a seat close to them.
- **Set up your table** exactly the same way you do while practising. Competition grounds are hardly places where you should try new things. A familiar setting of the table will help you stay organised and relaxed. You know where things are and won't panic while looking for them.
- **Prep your model if this is allowed.** Some competitions allow prepping the model's nails before the briefing, but some strictly prohibit that. Make sure that it's allowed before you start doing so, or else you may have points deducted. You could even be disqualified for that.
- **Prepare yourself and try to relax.** Listen to music, crack jokes with your model, talk to others, meditate, do whatever works for you as long it's legal and appropriate.
- **Don't pay attention to what others do**, stick to your routine and you'll be fine. Every tech has a different way of doing their work. Some polishes one hand just after buffing nails on the other, while another do that at the end. Stick to your way and focus on your models only.

- **Never touch the nails of other competitors' models**. Once the time is up you can have a look at them. However, never touch the models' hands or nails, you may be disqualified for that.
- **Remember you're there to compete against yourself and time!** You've made preparations and practised for long. Now is the time to shine forth!

Set your table:

- If you have a table to yourself you can use it the way you like. A common table would require you to respect the needs of other competitors, and don't take up too much space;
- use lint-free towel or bed coach to avoid fluff;
- use a dust collector if that's how you normally work;
- make sure you have all the products and tools needed on the table, as some competitions don't allow opening cases after the start.

Required products and stuff on the table:

- All products must be labelled, including water bottle/spray;
- sanitation products for skin and tools;
- filled-in client consultation form for your model;
- protection glasses and gloves.

Briefing (explanation of tasks and rules to all competitors) takes place 30-40 minutes before the competition begins. During that time you will not be allowed to touch your model's nails or leave the competition area. You may be disqualified if you don't follow these rules.

II. MODEL

Your model's role here is extremely important. She's not there just to "lend" you her nails and hands. She's also your motivator, fan, supporter and time-keeper. She provides that second pair of eyes, looking at the nails from a different viewpoint, i.e. from her side. Let's face it – your model is as crucial as your tools and skills.

She also has two more things to do – to make sure she's been judged and to shine next to you on the podium, if you make it. However, before I tell you more about it, let me say a few words about some seemingly insignificant things.

- If you've travelled with her then **arrive at the competition together;** if not, meet at the entrance. Just like you, she shouldn't be drinking too much water and soft beverages, as there'll be hardly any time for visiting ladies room during the competition and judging process.
- **It'll be very helpful if she wears a black top free from fluff**. A dark background sets off the nails and hands you're working on, and helps you focus your attention on them.
- **Keep her warm**. If she's cold then it may affect setting time if you're working with acrylic. Coldness will also turn her hands purple, which is not what the judges are looking for. You may lose points in overview, as frozen fingers never look as good as the warm ones.

- **Her hand must display the number tag all the time**. You'll be given a number at the registration desk. One sticker is for your model's hand and another is for you. None of you should remove them until the end of the event.
- **She may check the time for you**. Ask your model to do that. I like being told how much time is left, not gone, and I like to be told every 10-15 minutes.
- **She isn't allowed to leave the competition area until she's been judged**. This is your model's responsibility to see that she's been seen by all the judges and her nails have been marked. The number of judges may vary between three and six per category.
- **She mustn't allow anyone to touch her nails**. Other competitors or anyone else present would like to see her nails. This is absolutely normal, but she must protect them well to avert a possible disaster the nail polish may be still wet so touching would smudge them and you'd lose points.
- **She mustn't wear any jewellery.** Even wedding or engagement ring must be removed and tattoo, if any, covered.
- **This is unofficial;** she may help you with moisturising her cuticles by licking them. You'll see almost all of the models doing it while queuing up to be judged. Most of the competitions don't allow participants to use cuticle oil as treatment. No problem. You can still spruce up your model's cuticles with a wet cotton bud and ask her to moisturise them.

Judging rules and processes are always different. However, some rules are common across competitions.

- Judges are very focused. They will evaluate only the model's hands and nothing else.
- Models will be put in a numerical order and must present their hands to the judges.
- **The overview,** part one of the procedure, allows judges to set the standard for the competition with reference to the competitors' work. No detailed marking is done at this stage, only a general view is taken.
- Part two of the procedure is **proper judging**. Models will present their hands again, but this time every aspect of their nails will be marked in the score sheets in accordance with the standard.
- In case of a tie the affected models will be called back and their scores re-evaluated. Judges can also review marks, if unsatisfied.
- Models may leave only when they're asked to do so.

Awards ceremony for a particular category may take place the very same day the contest has been held under it, or on the last day of the competitions. Many competitors find waiting for the results more stressful than the contest. I'm one of them. Once the results are out, celebrate like there's no tomorrow. You've done something outstanding that only a few can match! Be proud of yourself!

EMERGENCY SITUATIONS

Emergency situations may arise and you should be well prepared to deal with them. I'm going to take you through the most common "situations" that I've experienced. I want you to remember that no matter what happens – there's always a solution. Remain calm and focus on finding a way out; and don't give up as long as you see a ray of hope.

FORGOTTEN PRODUCT OR TOOL

Imagine yourself in this situation you're at the competition venue busy setting up your table and getting ready mentally. As you start arranging all your products and tools on the table you notice you've forgotten something important! You start panicking and desperately look for a solution.

Keep calm! Panicking is not going to help here. You have several options depending on what you're missing:

- **Go and buy it** – if the competition takes place during a trade show, then it shouldn't be a problem for you to find a new one.

- **Borrow from someone** – fellow feeling will induce most of the competitors to come to your aid. It happened to me once. I forgot to get my buffers out of the beauty case and I wasn't allowed to open my case because the competition had already started. A girl sitting next to me had five buffers — one for two nails — and she loaned me her buffer each time she finished buffing two nails.
- **Ask the organiser or the floor judge to help**. It's unlikely that they'll have any stuff, but they can ask other competitors, who are sitting at a distance, to help you.
- **Can you work without it?** There are some tools that you can do without. If for example you've forgotten to take a 180-grit file with you, you can always use one with 150 or 100 grits. You'll end up having far more buffing to do, but it's still possible to finish on time.

Forgetting your products or tools can be very stressful. You can avert such a situation if you've followed my checklist to pack your case you'll have more stuff than necessary. Maybe someone else would need them. Winning competitions is great, but playing fair and helping others give you a greater win. Also remember what goes around, comes around.

MODEL DIDN'T SHOW UP

What could be worse than having no model to work on! This scenario is as bad as it sounds. It's quite simple to replace or borrow a product, but no one will share a model with you. It's definitely going to freeze or boil your blood, but again – think! There's always a way out.

If your model lets you down, here are your options:

- **Killing her later is definitely not one of them ;).**
- **Use your backup model**. Backup comes in handy when your main fails to turn up for whatever reason.
- **Use a friend**. If you arrive with a friend – male or female – use him/ her! At least you'll have some nails to work on!
- **No friend? Use a visitor.** In case you have nobody with you that day, ask anyone from the audience to be a model for you. Some would like to work for money while some others may just volunteer for you.

Whatever happens – don't give up! You may be stressed for not working on your model, but at least you're still in the game. You're a true fighter and that's what makes you a great person.

BROKEN NAIL

You may end up breaking a corner or the whole nail while filing or buffing to a high shine. Such an eventuality is quite common especially when nails are very thin. One uncontrolled move and it's gone. Always try to stick to the time allotted for each activity so you don't have to rush and do things, such as pulling corners too strong, in a hurry.

You may have the following situations to deal with:

- **Broken corner**:
  - If you have plenty of time left, you can remove the whole nail and do it from scratch;

- if you were elongating the nail bed then file off the free edge only and replace it;
- if you have very little time left then reapply the form and sculpt a new corner.

- **Broken nail**:

  - If you have time then remove the whole nail and do it all over again;
  - if you have not time then just glue it back.
  - if there's no time and you cannot use glue, use gel or acrylic to put it back on.

You will lose some points, but you'll also gain a few for a smile line, free edge shape etc.

Remember that glued back nails are far better than not having a full set done.

BLEEDING CUTICLE

Your model's cuticle may start to bleed, especially if you performed a full manicure the day before, or you're using her the same day in another category. It is highly likely that over-use may lead to such a situation because cuticles are very sensitive.

- Follow this step-by-step procedure, if that happens to you:
- Sanitise that area,
- press it firmly with a nail wipe,
- apply a small amount of nail glue to stop it from bleeding.

This is the fastest and easiest way to stop the bleeding and it allows you to keep working and not wasting too much time. If you don't to have the glue on your table, continue with pressing only and be extremely gentle when filing or buffing this nail.

SHORTER NAIL

Imagine you've filed all of the ten nails and you keep measuring them; and when you're doing the final check you find that one is too short! What can you do?

- If you have enough time you may shorten all nails, but that would mean re-shaping them all once more, as shortening will make them a hair line too thick.
- If it's not a significant difference then see that the shortened nail matches in measurement its counterpart on the other hand.
- Constantly measure the nails, as it saves you time and stress.

RUNNING OUT OF TIME

Most competitions expect you to do a set of nails on both hands in 2.5 hours. It's not a lot of time as it will quickly pass without you noticing it.

Once you've read the rules and judging criteria, you'll know how many points you're going to get for each segment. You should also realise that valuable points, which are so vital to your success, will be lost if you don't finish on time. Do stick to the time allotted to each exercise and have all the tasks done on time. The tasks might involve doing one hand or a number of nails if only one hand is meant to be done in pink and white and the second one polished in red. If you find yourself in a sticky situation where you don't have time to do everything you should, and where you have to choose between applying nail polish or shining the second hand – go for nail polish. Even though you will lose points for the lack of shine on one hand, you'll still gain some for the finished set and the nail polish. The scenario is bad enough, but it's better to finish a set, nail polish and all.

Whatever happens you must find a way to sort it out. In fact, you can always find one; so keep your cool, open up your mind and think. Don't hit the panic button. Every emergency situation teaches you some important lessons and makes you a better nail technician.

PART III

AFTER THE COMPETITION

Now is the time to relax. It's over but very few can actually heave a sigh of relief. Contestants wait with bated breath for the results to come in. Your hands get cold and clammy, you're so tense! Get yourself busy to ride out the trauma. Take lots of photos of your model's nails when she's back from the judges or else it may be too late. Nails break easily due to their thinness.

After the award ceremony you'll have more things to do. I'll talk about it soon, but for now I want to tell you this:

It doesn't matter if you're placed or not!
You win as long as you give hundred per cent!

Being placed is fantastic. Winning nothing creates an opportunity for you to shine better next time. I want you to remember the whole experience. Remember how much time and effort did preparation cost you? How many times did you have to say "NO" to something to focus on preparation and training? How disciplined and organised did you have to be? How did this whole experience change you as a person and make you a better nail technician? You were too scared to do this, but you did it. How much you've learnt!

At the end of the day, this is what really matters. You've gained more than just a trophy or a certificate. You've learnt how to play fair, push yourself hard and do things that seems impossible. In the industry, it will give you a far better position than that of your next-door rival. It will improve your CV and make you a much sought-after person. Benefits are endless not only for the winners, but also for everyone else who took part. It's your job to let people know that you've arrived and I'll tell you how to do that in a little while.

For now – let's talk about the other tasks that you've got to do once the competition's over.

FEEDBACK FROM THE JUDGES

One of the best things available to you as a competitor is the opportunity to speak to the judges after the awards ceremony. This is vital to your growth and learning as nail technician. Not many contestants use this opportunity to speak to the judges. But you should step forward and get informal feedback from all of the judges who were scoring your nails. Even if you have scored great marks there's always room for improvement. Ask them what could be improved, how to improve it and how to eliminate your mistakes. This feedback may help solve problems that have been nagging you for a while. It's also an important point of view from a person who knows what he/she is doing. He/she may be an industry veteran!

It may be a challenge to speak to all of the judges, as they usually don't stay around after the competition. Choose the one whose feedback you'd value most and rush to that person once the awards ceremony is over. You'll get first-hand info about how to improve your performance.

LEARN FROM YOUR MISTAKES ANALYSE YOUR SCORE SHEET

It's time to study the feedback that you've received from the judges or a judge and analyse the score sheet from the competition. The results show in black and white your strongest and weakest points. You may be very surprise once you see that. I was, when I got my first score sheet. It appeared that my strongest points were totally different from what I'd thought. One thing I want you to remember is that the points you've scored are specific to the competition you have participated in. The same performance in another competition would give you different scores!

You should pay a lot of attention to any score sheet of yours as it tells exactly what to do better next time to score higher.

Let me give you an idea of how to analyse the score sheet.

- If you were given 6 or less points, you have a lot to improve there. When practising for your next competition, focus on all areas with low scores as you need to work on these places.

- 7 – 8 points – Ok, You've got the skill, but your technique could be better and more consistent.
- 9 – It's a very good score meaning you're very close to perfection. Only small things need improvement.
- 10 – The highest point you can get. If you get ten you should be very proud of yourself as you've worked extremely hard and your work is flawless.

Nail competitions are all about gaining as many points as possible, so use every opportunity to improve your skills and techniques. It will require a lot of work, but it will also be rewarded. Play this game smartly. Play the nails game to win!

CAPITALISE ON YOUR WIN

You haven't thought that we're done, have you? Good, this is just the beginning of a new road that you need to travel. Now it's time to make the most of your win, or entry. It's time to talk business.

All the hard work you did, stress and strain you went through, and the great sense of elation you felt after winning the contest have finally led you to your final task of capitalising on it. What's the point of entering and winning a competition and keeping it to you? None! That's why I've asked Louise Prunty, proud winner of many business awards, to share with you her top tips and advice on how best to capitalise on your win.

Even if you're not a competition winner or you're not yet interested in contests, this information is still going to help you grow your business and promote it!

Bank on the press to share your success with people and keep them informed about the good work you do or the excellent services you offer. Let's say you're an educator and have a young student who is very passionate about the nail industry. She opens her own salon shortly and is doing really well. Isn't this success story worth publishing in local newspapers? A student of mine has a similar story.

You're not an educator but only a nail technician. Let's say you just finished a nail art course, or have learnt a new technique which is not very popular yet. It makes you quite unique in your area. Some PR with the press should be in order as you'd like to tell people that you supported charity and that a celebrity had visited in your salon and enjoyed your service.

Just as your job is to treat people with fantastic looking nails, journalists' job is to treat them with news! They have to write about something anyway, so why not to make them write about you and your business?

Enjoy the interview and learn as much as possible from it.

PRESS RELEASE WORTH PUBLISHING - AN EXCLUSIVE INTERVIEW WITH LOUISE PRUNTY

WHAT FOLLOWS AFTER THE COMPETITION?

"You are now an award winner! Congratulations. You may be asked to give a presentation, take special classes, write an article for a magazine or talk at events.

"My name is Louise Prunty, I have been in the beauty industry for ten years and I am the author of *How to Become an Award Winning Business in 7 Steps*.

"My companies have won many awards over the years and believe awards have had a crucial part to play in how people perceive us as a business. What you do after you've won an award is where the magic happens. If you do not promote your win you will not benefit from the world of opportunities that will unfold. So my advice is, **let everyone know about it.**

"This is not the end, this is not even the beginning of the end, this is just perhaps the end of the beginning."

—Winston Churchill

"Ensure you thank the event organisers in person and by email. Now get to work on your PR!

Some activities you can do include:

1. **Issuing a press release** to all relevant media in your industry plus a press release through a distribution service (examples of free PR submission websites:)
2. **Direct mail campaign** to your customers announcing the win and thanking them for their support.
3. **Promote yourself on social media**. Post to your accounts on Facebook, Twitter, Pinterest, etc., with a short message of your win plus a photograph.

   "If you have any Celebratory Offer/Award Win Offer, such as a special training day with you, "the award winning nail technician," or promotion of your new book etc., post it the following day as a limited space offer if it is a training course. Otherwise it can go as some kind of special one-off offer. Make sure you use social media and post on it regularly.
4. **Include the award logo** or words "Award Winning Nail Technician" on your email signature, letter head, web site and signage.
5. **Host a party or open day** with your staff, customers and possibly partners and suppliers to celebrate the win.

6. **Attach the words** "Award Winning" or an Award Winner logo to the new marketing material you develop.
7. **Keep the momentum going**, select the next award you are going to enter (even if it is months away), start your research and plan to win.

An award win is often an overlooked marketing tool which can take your company beyond the normal marketing routes."

PRESS RELEASE

The following press release is fictitious; it's just an example of the layout of a potential press release. You can use it as a template for your own. After you've written your press release, email it to all trade magazines that would be interested in your win.

You can use a press release distribution service to tap other media who'd like to receive and possibly publish your news. This will enable you to appear on Google as well. People looking for your name on the Net will come across the press release. (This can sometimes take some time to appear on Google).

FREE PRESS RELEASE DISTRIBUTION:

There are paid services for press release distribution but these are the free ones that I have found to be effective in reaching the right people.

http://www.prfire.co.uk/ UK Submission
http://bignews.biz/ USA Submission
https://www.pr.com/

Press release example:

FOR IMMEDIATE RELEASE

Date the press release to indicate when it's due; use the words IMMEDIATE RELEASE for recent and fresh events.

Nail Experts Academy Announces
Nail Technician Award Winner

Short, informative, eye-catching heading.

Summary

After a rigorous judging process the Nail Experts Academy Nail Technician of the Year has been chosen.

Students of Ela Loszczyk, founder of Nail Experts Academy, submitted their entries for the photographic competition. The standard for submissions was extremely high. However, a clear winner has emerged. Jane Smith is the overall winner and has bagged the title of –"Nail Technician of the Year".

Summarise the press release in this section. Journalists will read this part to see if the news is worth publishing.

About Nail Experts Academy

Our mission is to teach and help students at any level to realise their full potential so they become inspired and successful nail technicians and can live their passion.

Nail Experts Academy is an academy of the twenty-first century. We run live classes, but we focus on online and DVD training courses. This is how we can reach out to more students and nail technicians and help them learn new techniques.

Give additional details in this section of the press release.

About Jane Smith (Winner)

Jane Smith is a nail technician from Glasgow, Scotland. She has been working in the industry for only three years. In this short time she has developed her skills and become an outstanding technician/artist. She is a deserving winner of this award and her photos are world-class.

Review

"Jane is an inspiring individual, she is a determined lady and her dedication to the industry shows in her work"

Dean Harrod - DH Beauty

Jane is an outstanding nail artist, world-class work fit for the VOGUE magazine"

Lisa Tierney - Nail Academy - Surrey

Give any quotes or testimonials in this section.

END ###

NOTES TO EDITOR

Please contact Louise for any images or further information required.

PRESS RELEASE CONTACTS

Provide full address, telephone number

And email address.

END ### is the official way to end a press release.

NOTES & CONTACT DETAILS should be given.

Remember:

1: Do NOT attach images to the press release you are e-mailing. Spam filters of many companies will block e-mail messages with attachments, which means your press release will never be read. Always state that they can e-mail for images.
2: Try to keep your press release short and to the point. A two-page statement is perfect.
3: When someone does follow up on your press release make sure you respond immediately. Do not keep people waiting as they are likely to be working to a tight deadline.

BEHIND THE SCENES WITH ALEX FOX

Another treat is an exclusive interview with **Alex Fox** who's a Nailympian – an international competition organiser. She shared with me some behind-the-scenes facts about the competitions and I'm sure you're going to enjoy this highly motivational conversation.

WHAT'S THE STORY BEHIND NAILYMPIA AND HOW DID YOU GET INVOLVED?

This is the tenth year of my holding the international nail competition. Way back in 2000, when it was created by the heads of three USA manufacturers, EzFlow, IBD and Too Much Fun, I supported the concept and promoted it through a nail magazine I was then editing. This led to an invitation to travel to its home, Las Vegas, and help promote it further by covering it personally. The competition impressed me so much that I asked the organisers if I could run a sister competition in London. They said I could.

I modelled the London chapter on the USA event using its structure, rules and regulations, and awarding system. I also added a few features that, I think, made it more appealing to the European market. Flags and flowers were put on the nail desks and music was played to create a funky atmosphere. More features came later.

WHAT'S UNIQUE ABOUT THIS COMPETITION?

Nailympia prides itself on telling people that it provides an eclectic panel of judges consisting of nail experts drawn from all over the world. The true international character of the competition also provides a level playing field and brings stakeholders from all corners of the world together for the good of the industry. It is divided into three categories to appeal to a wider spectrum of participants. It has evolved with time and reflects through its categories the trend in the global nail industry.

HOW ARE THE JUDGES SELECTED, AND WHAT ARE THE CRITERIA?

People of good standing and reputation in the industry are invited as judges. They may be expert educators, manufacturers, innovators, former winners or leading lights in their home countries.

WHAT DO JUDGES LOOK FOR IN P&W CATEGORIES?

In the systems categories, the most critical thing the judges look for is consistency. The shape of the nail is not the key to winning a category contest. The smile lines of all the ten nails and the apex placement on every nail must look similar. From application to finishing, consistency should rule every aspect of the nail art. Participants can score great marks if they follow it.

WHY SHOULD ONE ENTER NAIL COMPETITIONS?

Entering a competition helps nail technicians improve their skills and be noticed. Their focused approach to it with regular practice, passion and dedication make them disciplined too. Practice leads to perfection of service and that helps their businesses. Clients and colleagues of such a technician get very excited at the prospects of their friend winning a medal or a trophy at the contest. A reward for hard work. Irrespective of the results, doing a competition itself creates great PR possibilities. The tech sends press releases to local newspapers and his/her services get promoted. Also, one can use social media to this effect. The networking possibilities are endless when a tech participates in an international event.

HOW TO MAKE THE MOST OF THE ENTRY/WIN TO BOOST BUSINESS AFTER THE COMPETITION?

Talk to your local media about your journey from salon desk to nail desk at an international nail competition. Make sure the media understands that around 22 countries will be represented and it will be an eclectic mix of nail experts from all over the world. Talk to trade magazines and get your work, salon, career profiled for industry awareness and kudos. Blog about your experience use your experience to guide others who may not be confident enough to do the competition circuit. If you win a contest you can be a mentor to those aspiring to compete.

CAN YOU REMEMBER ANY FUNNY OR SCARY INCIDENT THAT OCCURRED ON THE COMPETITION DAY?

Yes. Time ran out for me in a competition and my model missed her flight home to The Netherlands. That was a really difficult situation.

For Janine, my colleague, and me, the most difficult part is registering everyone on the first day as everyone shows up with their models in one huge mass of humanity, speaking many languages and we know we must process everyone as quickly as possible. We work it out strenuously every year and the comps generally start on time.

We are lucky that the nail industry is full of fantastic individuals looking to participate in a great event and that keeps the competition ticking.

WHAT IS THE FUTURE OF NAIL COMPETITIONS? HOW AND WHERE DO YOU SEE THEM SEVERAL YEARS FROM NOW?

They will get bigger and better. The categories will continue to change in keeping with trends in nail markets across the world. We will see more and more competitions emerging around the world and getting increasingly greater consumer recognition. People will be intrigued by what techs are creating and it's a matter of time before a nail competition makes it to mainstream television. Imagine a TV show where techs will be invited to show in real time what they can do to nails, armed with a few materials and an hour! Well, it's going to happen any day now.

FINAL WORD

WHAT SHOULD YOU DO NOW?

It's simple – you have to take action. If you've already entered competitions before and you won, then this book will guide you to further success. If you're, however, about to enter one or haven't got results yet, then you should learn, learn and learn.

Nail competition is not rocket science. You can easily learn how to play this game well. If you're serious about winning a contest, you'll have to work hard to upgrade your skills, to change your mindset, and to create a full package, the winning package. You're sure to win this game.

Think about driving and how you learnt it. Before you were driving around the city you had to learn the theory first. You had to know all the rules, traffic symbols, and things you'd do to avert accidents. Then you started driving on a small ground in a closed and safe area to make sure you can put the theory into practice. When you've done all that, you take your first city drive. It feels scary, but you still press ahead because you know that someone is sitting next to you to guide you whenever needed. You need this person's help to succeed and to be able to act despite your fears.

I've been *that* person for my students and I can do the same for you too. If you're looking for a coach, who will help you succeed, who will share all her knowledge and experience with you without holding anything back, then visit my website www.elaloszczyk.co.uk and check how we can work together to bring you closer to success.

IT'S YOUR TURN. It's time to take action now. Work hard, only then can you shine and enjoy the fruits of hard labour.

I wish you many wins and success and hope to work with you soon.

With love,
Ela